Per Bech

# The Bech, Hamilton and Zung Scales for Mood Disorders: Screening and Listening

A Twenty Years Update
with Reference to DSM-IV and ICD-10

Second Revised Edition

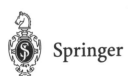

Springer

Per Bech, MD
Professor of Psychiatry
Frederiksborg General Hospital
Psychiatric Institute
Dyrehavevej 48
3400 Hillerød, Denmark

ISBN 3-540-61245-9 2nd Edition Springer-Verlag Berlin Heidelberg New York

ISBN 3-540-59104-4 1st Edition Springer-Verlag Berlin Heidelberg New York


With 2 Figures and 3 Tables

CIP-data applied for

Die Deutsche Bibliothek – CIP-Einheitsaufnahme
Bech, Per: The Bech, Hamilton and Zung scales for mood disorders: screening and listening:
a twenty years update with reference to DSM-IV and ICD-10 2nd edition / Per Bech. –
Berlin; Heidelberg; New York; London; Paris; Tokyo; Hong Kong; Barcelona; Budapest:
Springer, 1996
    ISBN 3-540-61245-9 (Berlin ...)

© Springer-Verlag Berlin Heidelberg 1996
Printed in Germany

Typesetting: K+V Fotosatz GmbH, Beerfelden, Germany
SPIN: 10536859        25/3134-5 4 3 2 1 0 – Printed on acid-free paper

A man looks up when he is
thinking of the future and down
when he is thinking of the past
*Aristotle*


When we first begin to
believe anything, what we
believe is not a single
proposition, it is a whole
system of propositions ...
Light dawns gradually
over the whole
*Wittgenstein*


There are very many different equally true
descriptions of the world ...
No one of these different descriptions is
*exclusively* true, since the others are also
true.
None of them tells us *the* way the world is,
but each of them tells us *a* way the world is
*Goodman*

# Preface

In no other group of medical disorders is it of greater importance, when establishing the patient-doctor collaboration, to make a proper screening interview, than it is in mood disorders. Doctor-rated interviews for mood disorders have been increasingly used over the last twenty years both in research and in the daily clinical work (not only in the psychiatric setting but also in general practice). The most widely used doctor-rated scale for depression, the Hamilton Depression Scale (HAM-D), has, over the last two decades, been revised for applicability in the various clinical settings. Questionnaires to be completed by the patients have been used to a much lesser extent. However, well-being questionnaires have recently been introduced into the medical setting as health-related quality of life instruments. The Zung Self-rating Depression Scale has often been used as model for well-being or quality-of-life questionnaires.

With the introduction in 1980 of the Diagnostic and Statistical Manual for Mental Disorders (DSM-III), mood disorders have been described by screening symptoms alone. Thus, the screening diagnosis of major depression according to the DSM-III system includes the same universe of symptoms as the HAM-D. However, the DSM-III symptoms are assessed only by dichotomies whereas the HAM-D symptoms are measured in degrees of severity.

When updating the scientific results with mood scales, the Hamilton and Zung Scales have been integrated with DSM-IV and ICD-10. One outcome of this approach is the Major Depression Rating Scale (with a DSM-IV as well as an ICD-10 version). Another outcome is the combined use of the WHO Well-Being Questionnaire and the Major Depression Rating Scale (Mastering Depression). This combination opens the patient-doctor collaboration. As a first step in treatment it shows for the patient that his or her doctor is familiar with the most frequent symptoms of mood disorders. In this stage of screening and listening the doctors and the scales indicate that they know the kind of feelings and thoughts that mood disorders bring to the patients.

Copenhagen, May 1996                                        Per Bech

# Contents

# 1 Introduction

The Hamilton Depression Scale (HAM-D [1]) is the scale most frequently used to measure the outcome of the acute treatment of depression. In this short-term treatment period the scale is more sensitive to reflecting changes in the depressive states than self-rating scales [2]. In a series of clinical trials with the HAM-D and global ratings in the late 1950's and the early 1960's it was found [3 – 5] that electroconvulsive therapy ECT was superior to imipramine in severely depressed inpatients (more than major depression), but that imipramine was superior to phenelzine in moderately depressed inpatients (major depression).

The impact of HAM-D on clinical psychiatry has been to promote the development of the syndrome approach to mental disorders, implying that no single symptom can be considered essential or necessary. The syndrome set of symptoms is considered sufficient if the items covary in a systematic way. Hamilton used factor analysis to test clinical syndromes [1].

The clinically most appropriate index of depression for studying the validity of a scale is a global clinical assessment performed by an experienced psychiatrist. The first study in this respect was the Danish study by Bech et al. [6]. The results showed that the HAM-D contained an index of depression which covered, however, only 6 of the 17 items. On the basis of this index and the Cronholm-Ottosson Depression Scale [7], the Melancholia Scale (MES) was developed [8]. Thus the MES should be considered as an index of the severity of depression. The MES is recommended for use in combination with the HAM-D when a multi-factorial approach (including anxiety and sleep factors) is essential, e.g. when measuring the profile of an antidepressant [9, 10]. See Appendix 1. For the measurement of antidepressive effect (including sensitivity in measuring improvement during treatment) the MES has been found superior to HAM-D [11, 12].

The diagnosis of depression (e.g. endogenous versus reactive melancholia) has been measured to a much lesser extent by rating scales than severity of depressive states. The most frequently used scale in this context has been the Newcastle (1965) depression scale [13], although the Newcastle (1971) version has also been used [10]. Both scales refer to one dimension only, with endogenous depression at one pole and reactive depression at the other. Eysenck [14] has criticised this one-dimensional approach, which implies that patients with mixed endogenous-reactive depression are insufficiently described. The Diagnostic Melancholia Scale (DMS) was developed from the two Newcastle scales and has two dimensions, one for endogenous depression and the other for reactive depression [15].

Hamilton did not develop a scale for mania because mania is a rare condition. However, in long-term treatment of depressive illness it is important to

**Internal validity**

− factor analysis
− latent structure analysis
 (Cronbach, Loevinger,
 Rasch)

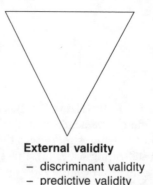

**Inter-rater reliability
or test − retest
reliability**

**External validity**

− discriminant validity
− predictive validity
− concurrent validity

**Fig. 1.** Triangle for analysis of screening scales

assess mania. The Bech-Rafaelsen Mania Scale [16] is one of the most frequently used scales for assessing manic or hypomanic symptomatology. In long-term trials with lithium or antidepressants it is recommended to use both the MAS and the MES. So far, however, the MES has been best analysed [17], e.g. in measuring relapse of depression (in this respect it has been found superior to HAM-D). Studies with the MAS in the prevention of relapse in manic states are in progress. The concordance between HAM-D, MES and DSM-III-R [18] or ICD-10 [19] has been described in detail elsewhere [10].

It is twenty years since Cochrane [20] published his small but significant book on effectiveness and efficiency in medicine. He described the screening test as the simplest possible diagnostic situation from which clinical research should always start. Statistically, he advocated for the use of univariate analysis to establish the point or points on the distribution scale of the screening symptom test at which therapy begins to do more good than harm, taking also into account the patient's point of view in the evaluation of the results of the screening test. He stated: "...A test is suitable as a diagnostic screening test if there is hard evidence, preferably based on randomized clinical trials.." [20].

Figure 1 shows the triangle for screening scales (as defined by Cochrane [20]) when psychometrically analysed for clinical meaning and communication. *Internal validity* refers both to the content validity of a scale (i.e. to what extent the items are representative of the clinical syndrome being analysed) and to the construct validity of the scale (i.e. to what extent the total score of the scale is a sufficient measure of the clinical syndrome). The two most frequently used models for testing internal validity are factor analysis and latent structure analysis (e.g. Loevinger's and Mokken's coefficient of homogeneity or Rasch analysis [10]).

*Reliability of communication* refers both to inter-rater reliability (i.e. to what extent different skilled observers (e.g. psychiatrists) agree when interviewing the same sample of patients) and to intra-patient reliability (i.e. to what ex-

**Table 1.** Standardization (external validity) of rating scales measuring the clinical dimensions of the four temperaments (melancholic, sanguine, choleric, and phlegmatic)

| Global assessment | | Depression categories | MES scores | Mania categories | MAS scores | Aggression categories | SDAS scores | Schizophrenia categories | BPRS scores |
| --- | --- | --- | --- | --- | --- | --- | --- | --- | --- |
| Categories | Scores | | | | | | | | |
| Normal | 0 | Melancholic temperament | 0 | Sanguine temperament | 0 | Choleric temperament | 0 | Phlegmatic temperament | 0 |
| Normal outliner | 1 | | 5 | | 5 | | 5 | | 5 |
| Mild | 2 | Hypothymia | 6 | Hyperthymia | 6 | Dysphoria | 6 | Borderline | 6 |
| | 3 | | | | | | | | |
| Moderate | 4 | Less than major | 14 | Hypomania | 14 | Passive aggression | 10 | Schizothymia | 14 |
| Moderate | 5 | Major depression | 15 | Mania | 15 | Violent acts predominantly verbal | 11 | Schizophrenia | 15 |
| Marked | 6 | | 25 | | 25 | | 17 | | 25 |
| | 7 | | | | | | | | |
| Severe | 8 | More than major depression (suicidal acts) | 26 | Psychotic mania | 26 | Violent acts, predominantly physical | 18 | Psychotic disintegration | 26 |
| | 9 | | | | | | | | |
| Extreme | 10 | | 44 | | 44 | | 36 | | 40 |

tent the patient gives consistent responses at different points in time; test – retest reliability or repeatability.

*External validity* refers to the clinical meaning of a scale. Predictive validity is the extent to which the scale can predict the outcome of treatment or relapse of illness. Discriminant validity refers to the extent to which a scale can differentiate between active and inactive treatment (responsiveness). Concurrent validity is the extent to which a scale correlates to other analogue scales, most frequently to a global clinical assessment performed by an experienced psychiatrist (often referred to as the standardization of a scale). Table 1 shows the standardization of scales measuring the four temperaments (melancholic, sanguine, choleric, and phlegmatic) with their corresponding clinical dimensions (depression, mania, aggression, and schizophrenia).

The triangle shown in Fig. 1 will be used to describe the screening dimension of a rating scale, i.e. its internal and external validity as well as its reliability.

The term "effectiveness" was defined by Cochrane [20]: "to measure the effect of a particular medical action in altering the natural history of a particular disease for the better by randomized clinical trials", and the term "efficiency" as: "to take the broad range of screening, place of treatment, rehabilitation, length of treatment, ... and quality of life into consideration". Furthermore, he concluded that the best example of therapies backed by randomized clinical trials is the drug therapy of tuberculosis whereas the worst example is in the area of antidepressants. He referred to the explanation given for this negative evaluation of antidepressants by Roth and Shapira [21], who had argued that the problem was due to the large numbers of other factors (social, personal, and genetic) which may affect the course of depressive illness.

This update of the rating scales for mood disorders is an attempt to show the psychometric developments in the spirit of Cochrane that have taken place over the last twenty years. Cochrane [20] made the suggestion both to increase the number of patients in randomized clinical trials with antidepressants and to increase the number of randomized clinical trials in order to achieve a proper meta-analysis. (The Cochrane Centre in Oxford [22] was established to produce systematic up to date reviews of all randomized clinical trials in health care.)

It is also twenty years since Feighner et al. [23] published the first major attempt to use screening diagnosis for symptoms alone in order to define mental disorders. A few years later the Research Diagnostic Criteria [24] was released, which provided the foundation for the third edition of Diagnostic and Statistical Manual for Mental Disorders (DSM-III). Both the DSM-III and its latest revision (DSM-IV [18]) have the screening diagnoses for mental disorders on axis 1. The screening diagnosis of major depression has been further developed for measuring outcomes of antidepressive therapies, the Major Depression Scale (see Appendix 3).

Attempts to going beyond the screening diagnosis of major depression have been made by using the other four DSM-III axes. The World Health Organization (WHO) has followed DSM-III and DSM-III-R in adopting the

**Table 2.** The multi-axial DSM-IV system in analysis of the screening diagnosis of major depression

| Axis 1 | Axis 2 | Axis 3 | Axis 4 | Axis 5 |
|---|---|---|---|---|
| (Major depression) | Neurotic personality | Secondary depression to somatic disorders | Reactive depression | Quality of life "disorders" |
| Consider biological symptoms:<br>– quality of depression<br>– late insomnia<br>– weight loss<br>– morning worst<br>– persistence of symptoms | – Eysenck's neuroticism | | Consider following symptoms<br>– reactivity of symptoms<br>– somatic anxiety<br>– long but fluctuating course | |

screening approach. Thus the tenth edition of the International Classification of Diseases (ICD-10) has been released [19] with screening diagnoses for mental and behavioural disorders. However, the multi-axial approach has so far not been released.

The combined use of the Hamilton Scales and the Newcastle Scales has shown how it is possible within the field of depression to go beyond the screening diagnoses of major depression by listening to the etiological or individual needs of the patient to be treated. Table 2 shows how the multi-axial principle in DSM-IV is used to separate endogenous depression from reactive depression. The Diagnostic Melancholia Scale (DMS) is described in Chap. 4.

Another way to progress beyond the screening diagnosis of major depression is to evaluate health-related quality of life factors. The multi-axial approach in DSM-III can be applied in the measurement of health-related quality of life (HRQL). Such scales measuring HRQL are described in Chap. 6. They were created by integrating the Zung Depression Scale, the WHO-TEN Scale and the PCASEE scale [10].

It is a century since Stanley Hall [25] published the first major study on the assessment of anger. He concluded his study by saying: "Probably our emotional psychology (melancholic, choleric, phlegmatic, sanguine) has now ... advanced to a stage ... (accepting that) the brain and not the heart (is) the general organ of mentation, and perhaps we are now at the dawn of a period of ganglionic psychology." Towards the end of this century we have unequivocal evidence that mood disorders are diseases of the brain. Thus the link between the somatic and emotional symptoms in the Hamilton Depression Scale is the brain. The psychometric clusters of symptoms covering melancholic, choleric and sanguine syndromes dealt with in this book underline the fact that mood disorders are diseases of the brain.

The term "major depression" was included in DSM-III to indicate the close association between this syndrome and interventions with antidepressant drugs. The term "major" goes back to DSM-II [26] in which "major affective disorders" was separated from neurotic affective disorders. Since 1980 around 85% of patients with major depression have been treated in the primary care settings. The Depression Guideline Panel [27] has listed the HAM-D, MES and the Montgomery Åsberg Scale among the rating scales for detection of major depression in the primary care settings. These scales are in the following described in the perspective of the primary care settings including mania and aggression scales within major affective (mood) disorders, but still maintaining construct validity: The focus is where the focus of correlation is [10, 28].

## References

1. Hamilton M (1960) A rating scale for depression. J Neurol Neurosurg Psychiatry 23:56–62
2. Edwards BC, Lambert MJ, Moran PW et al (1984) A meta-analytic comparison of the Beck Depression Inventory and the Hamilton Rating Scale for Depression as measures of treatment outcome. Br J Clin Psychol 23:93–99

3. Harris JA, Robin AA (1960) A controlled trial of phenelzine in depressive reactions. J Ment Sci 106:1432–1437
4. Robin AA, Harris JA (1962) A controlled comparison of imipramine and electroplexy. J Ment Sci 108:217–220
5. Robin AA, Langley GE (1964) A controlled trial of imipramine. Br J Psychiatry 110:419–422
6. Bech P, Gram LF, Dein E et al (1975) Quantitative rating of depressive states. Acta Psychiatr Scand 51:161–170
7. Bech P (1991) The Cronholm-Ottosson Depression Scale. The first depression scale designed to measure changes during treatment. Acta Psychiatr Scand 84:439–445
8. Bech P, Rafaelsen OJ (1980) The use of rating scales exemplified by a comparison of the Hamilton and the Bech-Rafaelsen Melancholia Scale. Acta Psychiatr Scand 62 [Suppl 285]:128–131
9. Bech P (1993) Acute therapy of depression. J Clin Psychiatry 54 [suppl 8]:18–27
10. Bech P (1993) Rating scales for psychopathology, health status and quality of life. Springer, Berlin Heidelberg New York
11. Maier W, Philipp M, Heuser I, Schlegel S, Buller R, Wentzel H (1988) Improving depression severity assessment. Reliability, internal validity and sensitivity to change of three observer depression scales. J Psychiatry Res 22:3–12
12. Lauritzen L, Bjerg Bendsen B, Vilmar T, Bjerg Bendsen E, Lunde M, Bech P (1994) Post-stroke depression: combined treatment with imipramine or desipramine and mianserin. A controlled clinical study. Psychopharmacology (Berl) 114:119–122
13. Carney MWP, Roth M, Garside RR (1965) The diagnosis of depressive syndromes and prediction of ECT response. Br J Psychiatry 111:659–674
14. Eysenck HJ (1970) The classification of depressive illness. Br J Psychiatry 117:241–250
15. Bech P, Allerup P, Gram LF et al (1988) The Diagnostic Melancholia Scale (DMS). Dimensions of endogenous and reactive depression with relationship to the Newcastle Scales. J Affective Disord 14:161–170
16. Bech P, Bolwig TG, Kramp P, Rafaelsen OJ (1979) The Bech-Rafaelsen Mania Scale and the Hamilton Depression Scale. Acta Psychiatr Scand 59:420–430
17. Lauritzen L, Odgård K, Clemmesen L et al (1996) Relapse prevention of paroxetine in ECT treated patients with major depression. A comparison with imipramine and placebo in medium-term continuation therapy. Acta Psychiatr Scand (in press)
18. American Psychiatric Association (1994) Diagnostic and statistical manual of mental disorders, 4th edn. (DSM-IV) American Psychiatric Association, Washington DC
19. World Health Organization (1993) The ICD-10 classification of mental and behavioural disorders. Diagnostic criteria for research. World Health Organization, Geneva
20. Cochrane AL (1972) Effectiveness and efficiency. The Nuffield Provincial Hospital Trust, London
21. Roth M, Shapira K (1970) Social implications of advances in psychopharmacology. Br Med Bull 26:197–202
22. Adams C, Gelder M (1994) The case for establishing a register of randomized controlled trials of mental health care. Br J Psychiatry 164:433–436
23. Feighner JR, Robins E, Guze SB, Wooddruff RA, Winokur G, Munoz R (1972) Diagnostic criteria for use in psychiatric research. Arch Gen Psychiat 26:57–63
24. Spitzer RL, Endicott J, Robins E (1978) Research Diagnostic Criteria. Arch Gen Psychiatry 35:773–782
25. Stanley Hall G (1898) A study of anger. Am J Psychology 10:516–591
26. Spitzer RL (1996) Where did "major depression" come from? Paper presented at the Major Depression Symposium, Copenhagen
27. Depression Guideline Panel (1993) Depression in primary care, 1: Detection and diagnosis. US Department of Health and Human Services, Rockville, Maryland (AHCPR publication 93-0550)
28. Loevinger J (1966) Psychological tests in the conceptual framework of psychology. In: Hammond KR (ed) The psychology of Egon Brunswik. Holt, Rinehart and Winston, New York, pp 107–148

# 2 The Bech-Rafaelsen Melancholia Scale (MES)

**Contents**

## 2.1 Scoring Sheet with Standardizations and DSM-IV/ICD-10 Criteria

| DSM-IV | No. | Item | Score | ICD-10 |
|---|---|---|---|---|
| 2 | 1 | Social life activities and interests | | A2 |
| 1 | 2 | Lowered mood | | A1 |
| 4 | 3 | Sleep disturbances | | B6 |
| | 4 | Anxiety | | |
| 2 | 5 | Introversion | | A2 |
| 8 | 6 | Concentration difficulties | | B4 |
| 6 | 7 | Tiredness | | A3 |
| 7 | 8 | Worthlessness and guilt | | B1,B2 |
| 5 | 9 | Decreased verbal activity | | B5 |
| 9 | 10 | Suicidal thoughts | | B3 |
| 5 | 11 | Decreased motor activity | | B5 |
| | | Total score | | |

The MES criteria (standardization) for total score:

| | |
|---|---|
| 0−5: | No depression |
| 6−9: | Mild depression |
| 10−14: | Less than major depression |
| 15−29: | Major depression |
| 30 or more: | More than major depression |

*The DSM-IV criteria for major depression:* Each of the nine DSM-IV items has a score of 1 if the corresponding MES item has a positive score. Major depression is then defined by a score of 1 on at least five of the nine items.

*The ICD-10 criteria for minor depression:* A score of 1 or more on two of three A items and on two of the seven B items.

*ICD-10 criteria for moderate depression:* A score of 1 or more on two of three A items and on four of the seven B items.

*ICD-10 criteria for severe depression:* A score of 1 or more on all three A items and on five of the seven B items.

## 2.2 Item Definitions

### General Remarks

The interview should assess the presence and intensity of the eleven items over a minimum period of three days. In many cases the last week is considered, and therefore, the time frame should be specified. During the interview it is not mandatory to follow the order of items as indicated in the scoring sheet, but experience has shown that the items follow each other in a logical way. However, the questions and the rank order will, of course depend on the condition of the patient. If the interviewer is in doubt in regard to an item, information should be solicited from relatives or, if the patient is hospitalized, from ward staff.

Since it has been observed in long-term studies of patients with manic-melancholic episodes that these states of mood are not necessarily mutually exclusive, it is possible for mixed states to develop. The combined use of the Melancholia Scale (MES) and the Mania Scale (MAS) has been recommended, especially in long term relapse-prevention or prophylactic therapies [1 – 3].

### Item Specifications

#### Item 1 Social Life Activities and Interests

Such activities and interests should be measured in terms of the degree of efficiency (performance and/or motivation) of the patient's functioning in social life, e.g. work, household tasks, school, leisure time, and structuring of daily activities in general.

0: No difficulties; feels time usefully spent.
1: Mild insufficiencies in social life activities; patient feels that he/she does not do enough social life activities.

2: Clear (little interest or pleasure in doing-things) but still only moderate insufficiencies in the patient's day-to-day activities.
3: Difficulties in performing even daily routine activities, which are carried out with great effort.
4: Often needs help in performing self care activities (unable to function independently).

### Item 2 Lowered Mood

0: Not present.
1: Slight tendency to lowered spirits.
2: The patient is more clearly preoccupied with unpleasant feelings although he or she still does not feel hopeless.
3: Markedly depressed. Some hopelessness and/or clear non-verbal signs of lowered mood.
4: Severe degree of lowered mood. Pronounced hopelessness.

### Item 3 Sleep Disturbances

This item covers the patient's subjective experience of the duration of sleep (hours of sleep per 24-h periods). The rating should be based on the three preceding nights, irrespective of the administration of hypnotics or sedatives. The score is the average of the past three nights.

0: Usual sleep duration.
1: Duration of sleep slightly reduced.
2: Duration of sleep clearly but still moderately reduced, i.e. still less than a 50% reduction.
3: Duration of sleep markedly reduced.
4: Duration of sleep extremely reduced, e.g. as if not been sleeping at all.

### Item 4 Anxiety

0: Not present.
1: Very mild tenseness, worry, fear or apprehension.
2: The patient is more clearly in a state of anxiety, apprehension or insecurity, which, however, he or she is still able to control.
3: The anxiety or apprehension is at times more difficult to control. On the edge of panic.
4: Extreme degree of anxiety, interfering greatly with the patient's daily life.

### Item 5 Emotional Introversion

0: Not present.
1: Very mild tendencies to emotional indifference in relation to social surroundings (colleagues).
2: The patient is more clearly emotionally introverted in relation to colleagues or other people but still glad to be with friends or family.

3: Moderately to markedly introverted, i.e. less need or ability to feel warmth toward friends or family.
4: The patient feels isolated or emotionally indifferent even to near friends or family.

### Item 6 Concentration Difficulties

0: Not present.
1: Very mild tendencies to concentration disturbances or problems in decision making.
2: Even with a major effort occasional difficulties in concentration.
3: Difficulties in concentration even in things that usually need no effort (reading a newspaper, watching television programme).
4: It is clear even during the interview that the patient has difficulties in concentration.

### Item 7 Tiredness

0: Not present.
1: Very mild feelings of tiredness.
2: The patient is more clearly in a state of tiredness or weakness, but these symptoms are still without influence on his/her daily life.
3: Marked feelings of tiredness which interfere occasionally with the patient's daily life.
4: Extreme feelings of tiredness which interfere more constantly with the patient's daily life.

### Item 8 Guilt Feelings

0: No loss of self-esteem, self-depreciation or guilt feelings.
1: The patients is concerned that he/she is a burden to the family, friends or colleagues due to reduced interests, introversion, low capacity or loss of self-esteem/self-confidence.
2: Self-depreciation or guilt feelings are clearly present because the patient is concerned with incidents (minor omissions or failures) in the past prior to the current episode of depression.
3: The patient feels that the current depression is a punishment but can intellectually still see that this view is unfounded.
4: Guilt feelings have become paranoid ideas.

### Item 9 Decreased Verbal Activity

0: Not present.
1: Very mild problems in verbal formulation.
2: More pronounced inertia in conversation, for example, a trend to longer pauses.
3: Interview is clearly coloured by brief responses or long pauses.
4: Interview is clearly prolonged due to decreased verbal formulation activity.

### *Item 10 Suicidal Thoughts*

0: Not present.
1: The patient feels that life is not worthwhile, but expresses no wish to die.
2: The patient wishes to die but has no plans taking his/her own life.
3: Probably has plans to hurt himself/herself.
4: Definitely has plans to kill himself/herself.

### *Item 11 Decreased Motor Activity*

0: Not present.
1: Very mild tendencies to decreased motor activity, for example, facial expression slightly retarded.
2: Moderately reduced motor activity, e.g. facial expression more clearly rigid, the head bent forward, looking down, reduced gestures.
3: Markedly reduced motor activity, e.g. all movements slow.
4: Severely reduced motor activity, approaching stupor.

## 2.3 Psychometric Description

*Type:* Symptom scale.

*Subject area:* Depression: severity of the illness and measuring change in depressive states during treatment.

*Administration:* Observer scale; semi-structured, goal-directed interview.

*Time axis:* The previous 72 h (minimum).

*Item selection:* Second generation scale based on those six valid items from the Hamilton Depression Scale that constituted an interval scale. Enlarged to include retardation items, such as emotional, intellectual, verbal, and motor retardation with reference to the Cronholm- Ottosson Depression Scale [4].

*Number of items:* 11.

*Definition of items:* All item definitions have operational criteria from 0 to 4.

*Psychometric validity:* Both internal and external validity indicate a general dimension for the severity of depression. Latent structure analysis (construct validity) shows that the scale is an interval scale [5 – 7]. When used in the elderly, factor analysis has confirmed that the MES items constitute one factor [8]. For standardization, see Table 1.

*Reliability:* Adequate inter-observer reliability has been found in several studies (around 0.80 in terms of intra-class correlation) [10, 11].

*Comments:* The pragmatic form of validity, which means that a new scale should have some practical advantages compared to existing scales, has been examined in studies by Schlegel et al. [12]. Thus the Melancholia Scale was found superior to the Hamilton Depression Scale in measuring psychomotor retardation, which was confirmed by the findings of Marcos and Salamero [8, 9]. The MES was found to be superior to the Montgomery-Åsberg Scale with respect to its sensitivity to measuring changes during treatment in severely depressed inpatients [5]. The predictive validity of the MES in chronic pain disorders in outpatient settings was found to be high by Loldrup et al. [13], who showed that the concept of less than major depression (scores between 10 and 14) predicts a good outcome for antidepressants. When combined with the Hamilton Scale (HDS/MES) the items cover both DSM-IV and the Montgomery-Åsberg Scale [14]. A self-rating version of MES [15] and structured interview have been developed [15]). The content validity of the MES is shown on the scoring sheet with reference to DSM-IV [16] and ICD-10 [17]. Recently a MES version which takes frequency and intensity measures into account has been released (see Appendix 2), especially for the assessment of recurrent brief depression [18]. This version (MES for Brief and Major Depression, MES/BMD) is applicable especially in depressions which are secondary to a medical illness. There have been made structured interviews for the MES, among them the Williams version [19] and the Smolka version [20]. The most systematic is the Smolka version which increases the inter-observer reliability from 0.80 to 0.91 in terms of intra-class coefficients. Smolka [20] showed furthermore, that the MES was very useful in the daily psychiatric routine when testing the quality of depression care.

The ability of the MES to detect depression in patients with medical complaints (e.g. pain disorders and stroke) is important because many depressed patients treated in primary care settings have medical co-morbidities [21]. In a recent study with post-stroke depression the MES was found more sensitive than HAM-D in measuring outcome of antidepressants [22].

## References

1. Bech P (1981) Rating scales for affective disorders. Their validity and consistency. Acta Psychiatr Scand 64 [suppl 295]:1 – 101
2. Bischoff R, Bobon D, Görtelmeyer R, Horn R, Müller AA, Stoll KD, Woggon B (1990) Rating scales for psychiatry: European edition. Beltz Test, Weinheim
3. Goodwin FK, Jamison KR (1990) Manic-depressive illness. Oxford University Press, New York
4. Bech P (1991) The Cronholm-Ottosson Depression Scale: the first depression scale to rate changes during treatment. Acta Psychiatr Scand 84:439 – 445
5. Maier W, Philipp M, Heuser I, Schlegel S, Buller R, Wetzel H (1988) Improving depression severity assessment. Reliability, internal validity and sensitivity to change of three observer depression scales. J Psychiatr Res 22:3 – 12
6. Maier W, Phillip M (1985) Comparative analysis of observer depression scales. Acta Psychiatr Scand 72:239 – 245
7. Chambon O, Cialdella P, Kiss L, Poncet F (1990) Study of the unidimensionality of the Bech-Rafaelsen Melancholia Scale (MES) using Rasch analysis in a French sample of major depressive disorders. Pharmacopsychiatry 23:243 – 245
8. Marcos T, Salamero M (1990) Factor study of the Hamilton Rating Scale for Depression and the Bech Melancholia Scale. Acta Psychiatr Scand 82:178 – 181

9. Lauritzen L, Odgård K, Clemmesen L et al (to be published) Relapse prevention of paroxetine in ECT treated patients with major depression. A comparison with imipramine and placebo in medium-term continuation therapy

10. Bech P, Gjerris A, Andersen J et al. (1983) The Melancholia Scale and the Newcastle Scales. Br J Psychiatry 143:58–63

11. Danish University Antidepressant Group (DUAG) (1990) Paroxetine: a selective serotonin reuptake inhibitor showing better tolerance, but weaker antidepressant effect than clomipramine in a controlled multicenter study. J Affective Disord 18:289–299

12. Schlegel S, Nieber D, Herrmann C, Bakauski E (1991) Latencies of the P 300 component of auditory event-related potential in depression are related to the Bech-Rafaelsen Melancholia Scale but not to the Hamilton Rating Scale for Depression. Acta Psychiatr Scand 83:438–440

13. Loldrup D, Langemark M, Hansen HJ et al (1991) The validity of the Melancholia Scale in predicting outcome of antidepressants in chronic idiopathic pain disorders. Eur Psychiatry 6:119–125

14. Kørner A, Nielsen BM, Eschen F et al (1990) Quantifying depressive symptomatology: inter-rater reliability and inter-item correlation. J Affective Disord 20:143–149

15. Bech P (1993) Rating scales for psychopathology, health status, and quality of life. A compendium on documentation in accordance with the DSM-III-R and WHO systems. Springer, Berlin Heidelberg New York

16. American Psychiatric Association (1994) Diagnostic and statistical manual of mental disorders, 4th edn. (DSM-IV) American Psychiatric Association, Washington DC

17. World Health Organization (1993) The ICD-10 classification of mental and behavioural disorders. Diagnostic criteria for research. World Health Organization, Geneva

18. Bech P (1993) Depressive syndrome in Parkinson's disease: clinical manifestations. In: Wolters EC, Scheltens P (eds) Mental dysfunction in Parkinson's disease. Vrije Universiteit Press, Amsterdam, pp 315–324

19. Williams JBW (1992) The structured interview for the Melancholia Scale. Biometric Research, New York State Psychiatric Institute

20. Smolka M (1995) Zur Evaluation der Bech-Rafaelsen Melancholie Skala. Dissertation, Freie Universität, Berlin

21. Depression Guideline Panel (1993) Depression in primary care, 2: Treatment of major depression. US Department of Health and Human Services, Rockville, Maryland (AHCPR publication 93-0551)

22. Lauritzen L, Bjerg Bendsen B, Vilmar T, Bjerg Bendsen E, Lund M, Bech P (1994) Poststroke depression: Combined treatment with imipramine or desipramine and mianserin. A controlled clinical study. Psychopharmacology (Berl) 114:119–122

# 3 The Bech-Rafaelsen Mania Scale (MAS)

**Contents**

## 3.1 Scoring Sheet with Standardiaztions and DSM-IV/ICD-10 Criteria

| DSM-IV | No. | Item | Score | ICD-10 |
|--------|-----|------|-------|--------|
| A1 | 1 | Elevated mood | | A1 |
| B3 | 2 | Talkativeness (pressure of speech) | | B2 |
| B6 | 3 | Increased social contact | | B4 |
| B6 | 4 | Increased motor activity | | B1 |
| B2 | 5 | Sleep disturbances | | B5 |
| B5 | 6 | Social activities (distractability) | | B7 |
| A2 | 7 | Hostility, irritable mood | | A2 |
| B7 | 8 | Increased sexual activity | | B9 |
| B1 | 9 | Increased self-esteem | | B6 |
| B4 | 10 | Flight of thoughts | | B3 |
| | 11 | Noise level | | |
| | | Total score | | |

The MAS criteria (standardization) for total score:

| | |
|---|---|
| 0–5: | No mania |
| 6–9: | Hypomania (mild) |
| 10–14: | Probable mania |
| 15 or more: | Definite mania |

*The DSM-IV criteria for mania:* If A2 is scored higher than A1, a manic classification requires at least four B items. If A1 is scored higher than A2, only three B items are needed.

*The ICD-10 criteria for mania:* If A2 is scored higher than A1, a manic classification requires at least four B items. If A1 is scored higher than A2, only three B items are needed.

## 3.2 Item Definitions

### General Remarks

The interview should assess the presence and intensity of the eleven items over a minimum period of the preceding 3 days. In many cases the last week is considered and therefore the time frame should be specified. During the interview it is not mandatory to follow the order of items as indicated on the scoring sheet but this order has been suggested because the items with the lowest number are the most inclusive, i.e. they are present even in minor degrees of mania (hypomania). When the interviewer is in doubt about an item, information should be solicited from relatives or, if the patient is hospitalized, from ward staff.

### Item Specifications

#### *Item 1 Elevated Mood*

0: Not present.
1: Slightly elevated mood, optimistic, but still adapted to situation.
2: Moderately elevated mood, joking, laughing, however, somewhat irrelevant to situation.
3: Markedly elevated mood, exuberant both in manner and speech, clearly irrelevant to situation.
4: Extremely elevated mood, quite irrelevant to situation.

#### *Item 2 Talkativeness (Pressure of Speech)*

0: Not present.
1: Somewhat talkative.
2: Clearly talkative, few spontaneous intervals in the conversation, but still not difficult to interrupt.
3: Almost no spontaneous intervals in the conversation, difficult to interrupt.
4: Impossible to interrupt, dominates the conversation completely.

## *Item 3 Increased Social Contact (Extraversion)*

0: Not present.
1: Slightly meddling (putting his/her oar in), slightly intrusive.
2: Moderately meddling and arguing or intrusive.
3: Dominating, arranging, directing, but still in context with the setting.
4: Extremely dominating and manipulating, not in context with the setting.

## *Item 4 Increased Motor Activity*

0: Not present.
1: Slightly increased motor activity (e.g. some tendency to lively facial expression).
2: Clearly increased motor activity (e.g. lively facial expression, not able to sit quietly in chair).
3: Excessive motor activity, on the move most of the time, but the patient can sit still if urged to (rises only once during interview).
4: Constantly active, restlessly energetic. Even if urged to, the patient cannot sit still.

## *Item 5 Sleep Disturbances*

This item covers the patient's subjective experience of the duration of sleep (hours of sleep per 24-h periods). The rating should be based on the three preceding nights, irrespective of the administration of hypnotics or sedatives. The score is the average of the past three nights.

0: Not present (habitual duration of sleep).
1: Duration of sleep reduced by 25%.
2: Duration of sleep reduced by 50%.
3: Duration of sleep reduced by 75%.
4: No sleep.

## *Item 6 Social Activity (Distractability)*

Social activity should be measured in terms of the degree of disability or distractability in social, occupational or other important areas of functioning.

0: No difficulties.
1: Slightly increased drive, but work quality is slightly reduced as motivation is changing; the patient is somewhat distractible (attention drawn to irrelevant stimuli).
2: Work activity clearly affected by distractibility, but still to a moderate degree.
3: The patient occasionally loses control of routine tasks because of marked distractibility.
4: Unable to perform any task without help.

### Item 7 Hostility

0: Not present.
1: Somewhat impatient or irritable, but control is maintained.
2: Moderately impatient or irritable. Does not tolerate provocations.
3: Provocative, makes threats, but can be calmed down.
4: Overt physical violence; physically destructive.

### Item 8 Increased Sexual Activity

0: Not present.
1: Slight increase in sexual interest and activity, for example, slightly flirtatious.
2: Moderate increase in sexual interest and activity, for example, clearly flirtatious.
3: Marked increase in sexual interest and activity; excessively flirtatious.
4: Completely preoccupied by sexual interests.

### Item 9 Increased Self-Esteem

0: Not present.
1: Slightly increased self-esteem, for example, overestimates slightly own habitual capabilities.
2: Moderately increased self-esteem, for example, overestimates more clearly own habitual capabilities or hints at unusual abilities.
3: Markedly unrealistic ideas, for example, believes he/she possesses extraordinary abilities, powers or knowledge (scientific, religious etc), but can quickly be corrected.
4: Grandiose ideas which cannot be corrected.

### Item 10 Flight of Thoughts

0: Not present.
1: Somewhat lively in descriptions, explanations and elaborations without losing the connection with the topic of the conversation. The thoughts are thus still coherent.
2: The patient's thoughts are occasionally distracted by random associations (often rhymes, slangs, puns, pieces of verse or music).
3: The line of thought is more regularly disrupted by diversionary associations.
4: It is very difficult or impossible to follow the patient because of the flight of thoughts; he or she constantly jumps from one topic to another.

### Item 11 Noise Level

0: Not present.
1: Speaks somewhat loudly without being noisy.
2: Voice discernible at a distance, and somewhat noisy.

3: Vociferous, voice discernible at a long distance, is markedly noisy or singing.

4: Shouting, screaming; or using other sources of noise due to hoarseness.

## 3.3 Psychometric Description

*Type:* Symptom scale.

*Subject area:* Mania: severity of the manic disorder, the screening approach, and detecting change during treatment.

*Administration:* Observer scale. Semi-structured, goal-directed interview [1, 2].

*Time axis:* The previous 72 h (minimum).

*Item selection:* Second generation scale, which was developed on the basis of an item analysis of Biegel's [2] nurse-administered scale for manic states and as a counterpart to the Melancholia Scale (MES).

*Number of items:* 11.

*Definition of items:* All items are defined according to operational criteria from 0 to 4.

*Psychometric validity:* Both internal and external validity indicate that there is a general dimension of mania. Loevinger's coefficient of homogeneity has been found to be 0.58 (acceptable) and Cronbach's alpha to be 0.93 [3]. For standardization, see Table 1.

*Reliability:* Inter-observer reliability in terms of intra-class correlation is 0.98.

*Comments:* The Mania Scale has been used in several clinical studies to evaluate the antimanic effects of lithium and ECT [4], carbamazepine [5], haloperidol [6], clonidine [7] and zuclopenthixol [8, 9]. In these studies the scale has been found to be sensitive to measurement changes during treatment. A self-rating version of MAS has been developed [3]. The content validity of the MAS is shown on the scoring sheet with reference to DSM-IV [10] and ICD-10 [11]. The MAS should be used in combination with SDAS-9 if assessment of aggression or hostility is needed, and possibly, with the BPRS psychotic disintegration scale if a dimension of psychosis is needed, e.g. in antipsychotic trials [12].

## References

1. Bech P, Bolwig TG, Kramp P, Rafaelsen OJ (1979) The Bech-Rafaelsen Mania Scale and the Hamilton Depression Scale. Acta Psychiatr Scand 59:420–430
2. Bech P (1981) Rating scales for affective disorders. Their validity and consistency. Acta Psychiatr Scand 64 [Suppl 295]:1–101

3. Bech P (1993) Rating scales for psychopathology, health status, and quality of life. A compendium on documentation in accordance with the DSM-III-R and WHO systems. Springer, Berlin Heidelberg New York
4. Small JG, Klapper MH, Kellams JJ et al (1988) Electroconvulsive treatment compared with lithium in the management of manic states. Arch Gen Psychiatry 45:727–732
5. Lusznat RM, Murphy DP, Nunn CMH (1988) Carbamazepine vs. lithium in the treatment and prophylaxis of mania. Br J Psychiatry 153:198–204
6. Gjerris A, Bech P, Broen-Christensen C et al (1981) Haloperidol plasma levels in relation to antimanic effect. In: Usdin E, Dahl SG, Gram LF, Lingjærde O (eds) Clinical pharmacology in psychiatry. McMillan, London, pp 227–232
7. Hardy MC, Lecrubier Y, Widlöcher D (1986) Efficacy of clonidine in 24 patients with acute mania. Am J Psychiatry 143:1450–1455
8. Amdisen A, Nielsen MS, Dencker SJ et al (1987) Zuclopenthixol acetate in Viscoleo R – an new drug formulation in patients with acute psychoses including mania. Acta Psychiatr Scand 75:99–107
9. Kørner A, Pedersen V, Bech P (1993) A meta-analysis of the anti-psychotic and anti-manic effects of zuclopenthixol acetate. Paper presented at the 9th World Congress of Psychiatry, Rio de Janeiro, 6–12 June
10. American Psychiatric Association (1994) Diagnostic and statistical manual of mental disorders, 4th edn. (DSM-IV) American Psychiatric Association, Washington DC
11. World Health Organization (1993) The ICD-10 classification of mental and behavioural disorders. Diagnostic criteria for research. World Health Organization, Geneva
12. Gouliaev G, Licht RW, Vestergaard P et al. (1996) Treatment of manic episodes: Zuclopenthixol and clomazepam versus lithium and clomazepam. Acta Psychiatr Scand 93:119–124

# 4 The Social Dysfunction and Aggression Scale (SDAS-9)

**Contents**

## 4.1 Scoring Sheet with Standardizations

| No. | Item | Score |
|-----|------|-------|
| 1 | Irritability | |
| 2 | Negativism/uncooperative behaviour | |
| 3 | Dysphoric mood | |
| 4 | Socially disturbing/provocative behaviour | |
| 5 | Non-directed verbal aggression | |
| 6 | Directed verbal aggression | |
| 7 | Physical violence towards things | |
| 8 | Physical violence towards staff members | |
| 9 | Physical violence towards non-staff | |
| | Total score | |

The SDAS criteria (standardization) for total score:

    0−5: No aggression
    6−10: Passive aggression
  11−17: Verbal acts of aggression
  18−36: Physical acts of aggression

## 4.2 Item Definitions

### General Remarks

The assessment of outward aggressiveness covers as a minimum period the preceding 3 days. The information to be considered depends greatly on the observations made by the staff members or reports by primary care workers or family. However, interpersonal behaviour observed during the interview is also important.

The items of the scale can be assessed both as the general level of outward aggression or hostility during the last 3 days and as the peak level (i.e. incidents or attacks of aggression). Within mood disorders it is important to measure outward aggression in manic states, and in these states generalized levels of hostility are most often seen. Therefore, only the generalized version of SDAS-9 is included here.

### Item Specifications

#### Item 1 Irritability

This item covers the reduced ability to cope with situations regarded as provocative by the patient, impatience, and the reduced ability to control responses. In other words, irritability is directed towards situations perceived as provocative by the patient.

0: Not present.
1: Slight or possible impatience and/or slight difficulty in controlling responses.
2: Mildly impatient and irritated; some difficulty in controlling reactions.
3: Moderately impatient, easily provoked, poor control over reactions, but this still has limited impact on personal relations.
4: Severe impatience and irritability, no control over reactions, feels constantly provoked which interferes significantly with interpersonal relations.

#### Item 2 Negativism/Uncooperative Behaviour

Covers the reduced ability to cooperate or to conform to a group, e.g. refuses to comply with ward regulations or management plan.

0: Not present.
1: Slight or possible opposition when discipline is required.
2: Mild negativism. Does not want to cooperate, e.g. refuses to perform a necessary task, but can control him-/herself when told to conform.
3: Moderate negativism: clearly obstructing all authority, though still moderate; sometimes undisciplined.
4: Severe negativism: ostentatious in opposing the rules of social intercourse; fully uncooperative.

### Item 3 Dysphoric Mood

Covers a general or indirect mood where the patient is dissatisfied, moody, testy, and fed up.

0: Not present.
1: Slight, or possibly present.
2: Mild; the patient has displayed a slight mood of dissatisfaction.
3: Moderate; the patient has given the impression of being moderately gloomy and testy but still with limited impact on interpersonal relations.
4: Severe; the patient has given the impression of being extremely sullen and crabby, displaying clear signs of intense discontent and dissatisfaction which significantly interfere with interpersonal relations.

### Item 4 Socially Disturbing/Provocative Behaviour

The patient behaves in a provocative manner towards others. This also includes sexually provocative behaviour.

0: Not present.
1: Slight, or possibly present.
2: The patient has acted provocatively, to a mild degree.
3: The patient has acted provocatively, to a moderate degree.
4: The patient has acted provocatively to a serious degree.

### Item 5 Non-directed Verbal/Vocal Aggressiveness

This item covers verbal aggressiveness or noises assumed to represent aggression which (instead of being directed towards defined persons) is directed towards people or things in general, e.g. the staff, the ward, or society in general.

0: Not present.
1: Very slight or possible verbal aggressiveness, though only implicitly present.
2: Mild aggressiveness which is explicitly present, but only intermittently.
3: Moderate level of verbal aggressiveness, sometimes vociferous, e.g. claiming "everything to be wrong" or shouting angrily.
4: Severe and sometimes screaming aggressiveness of general nature; this may include cursing or sweating.

### Item 6 Directed Verbal/Vocal Aggressiveness

Covers verbal aggressiveness directed towards particular people.

0: Not present.
1: Very slight or possible aggressiveness towards defined individuals.
2: Mild aggressiveness manifested by an explicit way of talking, though the aggressive contents are only present in short outbursts.
3: Moderate aggressiveness, e.g. insulting people personally, more constant, sometimes vociferous.

4: Severe and sometimes screaming aggressiveness, e.g. making serious insults or wishing people harm.

### Item 7 Physical Violence Towards Things

0: Not present.
1: Slight, or possibly present (threatening gestures).
2: Mild, occasional episode of throwing or hitting things.
3: Repeated episodes of throwing trivial things, hitting objects or slamming doors.
4: Severe, has been destroying large or important objects, i.e. TV, windows and furniture.

### Item 8 Physical Violence Towards Staff

0: Not present.
1: Slight, or possibly present (threatening gestures).
2: Mild: the patient has tried to hit out at/kick a member of staff. No severe injuries.
3: Moderate: the patient has kicked/punched a member of staff. No severe injuries.
4: Severe: the patient has dangerously assaulted a member of staff and/or has tried to strangle a member of staff.

### Item 9 Physical Violence Towards Others Than Staff (Non-staff)

For example, visitors or other patients.

0: Not present.
1: Slight, or possibly present (threatening gestures).
2: Mild: the patient tried to hit out at/kick non-staff, though without touching the person.
3: Moderate: the patient has kicked/punched non-staff. No severe injuries.
4: Severe: the patient has dangerously assaulted non-staff, and/or has tried to strangle non-staff.

## 4.3 Psychometric Description

*Type:* Symptom scale.

*Subject area:* Outward aggression considered as a generic (non-disease specific) dimension. However, in the context of mood disorders outward aggression is associated with mania.

*Administration:* Observer scale based on reports from staff members, primary care workers or family members.

*Time Axis:* The last 3 days (minimum).

*Item selection:* First generation scale based on the literature and comprehensive rating scales, especially the AMDP [1] and the Buss model of aggression [2, 3].

*Number of items:* Nine.

*Definition of items:* All items are defined according to operational criteria from 0 to 4.

*Psychometric validity:* The scale has been psychometrically validated in three studies: on non-organic disorders [4, 5] and on dementia and mental handicap [6]. The scale showed acceptable applicability in this condition, and the construct validity (Cronbach, Loevinger and Rasch analyses) was found to be adequate. For standardization, see Table 1.

*Reliability:* Inter-observer reliability in terms of intra-class correlation was also found acceptable [4, 5].

*Comments:* The SDAS-9 should be used in combination with the Mania Scale in trials with antimanic therapies because aggression is an important aspect of manic states. (In trials with dementia and mental handicap the SDAS-9 is recommended, especially for the peak assessment, because social dysfunction and aggression is often the focus of care in these states.) However, the psychotic disintegration scale may also be used in antipsychotic trials in combination with MAS and SDAS-9. The SDAS-9 has recently been shown to have a high degree of responsiveness during treatment with neuroleptics in schizophrenic patients [7], but also with the selective serotonin against eltoprazine [8].

# References

1. Ban TA, Guy W (eds) (1982) The manual for the assessment and documentation of psychopathology (AMDP System). Springer, Berlin Heidelberg New York
2. Buss AH (1971) Aggression pays. In: Singer JL (ed) The control of aggression and violence. Academic Press, New York, p8
3. Bech P (1994) Measurement by observations of aggressive behaviour and activities in clinical situations. Crim Beh Ment Health. 4:290–252
4. Wistedt B, Rasmussen A, Pedersen L, Malin U, Träskman-Bendz L, Berggren M, Wakelin J, Bech P (1990) The development of an observer scale for measuring social dysfunction and aggression (SDAS). Pharmacopsychiatry 23:249–252
5. European Rating Aggression Group (ERAG) (1992) Social dysfunction and aggression scale in generalized aggression and in aggressive attacks. A validity and reliability study. Int J Method Psychiatr Res 1992 2:15–29
6. Bech P, Mak M, Pedersen L and the ERAG (to be published) The applicability and validity of social dysfunction and aggression scale in patients with dementia and mental handicap in comparison with patients with functional mental disorders
7. Bang-Kittilsen A, Asserson S, Elgew K (1995) Kvalitetskontroll av zyclopenthixol acetat has psykotiske patienter med aggressiv holdning eller adford (quality of care in psychotic patients with aggressive behaviour treated with zyclopenthixol). Nordic J Psychiatry 49 (Suppl 35):79–93
8. Tiihonen J, Hakola P, Paanila J, Turtianinen M (1993) Eltoprazine for aggression in schizophrenia and mental retardation. Lancet 341:307–308

# 5 The Diagnostic Melancholia Scale (DMS)

**Contents**

## 5.1 Scoring Sheet with Standardizations

Endogenous Melancholia

| No. | Item | Score |
|-----|------|-------|
| E1 | Quality of depression | |
| E2 | Early awakening | |
| E3 | Weight loss | |
| E4 | Diurnal variation, morning worse | |
| E5 | Persistence of clinical picture | |
| Total score | | |

Reactive Melancholia

| No. | Item | Score |
|-----|------|-------|
| R1 | Psychological stressors | |
| R2 | Reactivity | |
| R3 | Somatic anxiety | |
| R4 | Duration of episode | |
| R5 | Character neurosis | |
| Total score | | |

The DMS criteria (standardization) for total score:

E $(1-5) \geqslant 5$ and R $(1-5) < 5$: endogenous melancholia
E $(1-5) < 5$ and R $(1-5) \geqslant 5$: reactive melancholia
E $(1-5) \geqslant 5$ and R $(1-5) \geqslant 5$: mixed endogenous/reactive melancholia

## 5.2 Item Definitions

**General Remarks**

As formulated by Wing [1], to put forward a diagnosis is, first of all, to recognize a condition, i.e. the screening approach, and then to put forward a theory about it. The Melancholia Scale (MES) is a screening tool for recognizing depressive illness which in terms of the MES criteria can be placed on the spectrum of mild, less than major, major, and more than major depression or melancholia. (It should be emphasized that melancholia according to Hamilton [2] refers to depressive illness and not to a diagnosis in itself which unfortunately is the case in DSM-IV [3].)

The most valid theories for melancholia are the biological approach included in the term "endogenous depression" [4] and the psychological approach included in the term "reactive melancholia" [5]. The Diagnostic Melancholia Scale (DMS) has a dimension both for endogenous (items E1 to E5) and for reactive (items R1 to R5) melancholia. It has been found that the two dimensions are not mutually exclusive, hence the term "mixed endogenous and reactive melancholia".

The components relevant for the dimensions of endogenous and reactive melancholia are, to a certain extent, the DSM-IV axes of mental symptoms, personality issues, somatic symptoms, psychosocial stressors, and social functioning. However, social functioning is an indicator of the severity of illness, not a diagnostic indicator. Furthermore, in depressive illness the course of symptoms has in itself a diagnostic impact, e.g. diurnal variation, morning worse; reactivity, persistence and duration of symptoms [6, 7].

Against this background the DMS should be measured after the MES assessment and should take into account the current episode as well as the personality traits.

In contrast to the MES, in which each item is anchored from 0 (not present), 1 (mild), 2 (moderate), 3 (marked), to 4 (very severe), the DMS items are anchored from 0 (not present), 1 (mild or probable), to 2 (clear or definite). The domain of each DMS item has been defined in detail as follows:

**Item Specifications**

*Item E1 Quality of Depression*

This item covers the patient's experience of the current depressive episode as qualitatively distinct from normal despondency when under adversity or distress, e.g. the death of a loved one. Therefore, the patient should be asked about qualitative feelings different from the range of his ordinary affective responses to distress. It is a difficult item to assess, especially, of course, if the patient denies ever having had severe distress. It is of importance to ascertain whether prior to the current depressive episode, i.e. in his habitual state, the patient has experienced the same kind of symptoms as now, or whether the current symptoms are more of a "foreign body", a distinct quality of depression.

0: The current depressive episode has been described as "ordinary" sadness as experienced in adverse situations such as death in the family or circle of friends.
1: The interviewer or the patient is in doubt as to the quality of the experience.
2: The patient cannot identify himself with the current depressive syndrome, which therefore is conceived as qualitatively distinct from feelings of grief.

### Item E2 Early Awakening

Early awakening refers to the patient waking up at least 1 hour earlier than usual. The assessment of this item should include the general (average) sleep pattern during the current depressive episode, and not only the previous days. (Disregard whether the patient has been using sedative/hypnotic medication.)

0: No early awakening.
1: Doubtful or the patient has had this symptom only during the past few days.
2: The interviewer is convinced that a persistent feature during the present episode the patient has woken up at least 1 h too early.

### Item E3 Weight Loss

0: No weight loss related to the current episode.
1: A less pronounced weight loss.
2: The patient indicates a weight loss of 3 kg or more related to the current depressive episode, or 0.5 kg or more per week during the past 3 weeks.

### Item E4 Diurnal Variation

Diurnal variation means that during the current depressive episode the patient has generally (on average) been most depressed in the morning hours, and that the severity of depression diminishes during the day. The criterion for diurnal variation is not fulfilled if the patient indicates only a brief improvement just before going to bed.

0: There is no diurnal rhythm.
1: It is doubtful whether a truly autonomous diurnal variation is present.
2: The interviewer is convinced that during the current episode the patient has a diurnal rhythm in the severity of his symptoms. (Take habitual diurnal variation and possible reactivity into account.)

### Item E5 Persistence of Clinical Picture

This item refers to the clinical picture, the depressive syndrome, being in general constant during the current episode, apart from minor day-to-day variations and/or diurnal variation.

0: There have been clear fluctuations.
1: It is doubtful whether the clinical picture of the current episode is persistent.
2: There has been no significant change (fluctuations between "good" and "bad" days or weeks).

### Item R1 Psychological Stressors

Psychological stressors are all situations or events considered by the interviewer to have contributed significantly to the development of the current depressive episode. The stressors must have appeared within the 6 months prior to this episode and may or may not still be present and maintaining the depressive syndrome. The stressors may be worries concerning the patients's health, the health of near relatives or friends, the death of a loved one, interpersonal conflicts in the family or at work, or financial problems. The same stressor may, of course, be a very different experience for different patients, and the patient's subjective experiences and feelings must be taken into consideration. However, the interviewer's evaluation is decisive.

0: Psychological stressors have not been present.
1: The interviewer is in doubt.
2: Psychological stressors have been or are still present.

### Item R2 Reactivity of Symptoms

Reactivity means that the severity of the depressive symptoms waxes and wanes in relation to circumstances; for example, the patient feels less depressed when something pleasant or positive appears or takes place. The patient thus retains the capacity to react positively when something positive takes place or to feel less depressed for a while in good company.

0: There is lack of reactivity to usually pleasurable stimuli, that is, the patient does not feel much better, even temporarily, when something good happens.
1: Reactivity is only transient.
2: The interviewer is convinced that reactivity is present.

### Item R3 Somatic Anxiety

Somatic anxiety should be assessed independently of psychic anxiety. Somatic anxiety includes all physiological concomitants of anxiety: motor tension and autonomic hyperactivity (especially palpitations, nausea or vomiting, sweating, and dizziness). It is often difficult to distinguish between somatic anxiety and psychomotor agitation, but in this connection it is immaterial whether agitation is included in the score. It is also immaterial to distinguish between attacks of somatic anxiety and generalized anxiety. However, it is, decisive to assess whether during the current depressive episode the patient has experienced somatic anxiety, and the past week should be stressed most.

0: The patient has not experienced somatic anxiety.
1: In doubt.
2: During the past week and/or at the interview the patient has been clearly anxious (experienced motor tension, palpitations, nausea, sweating, etc.).

### Item R4 Duration of Current Episode

Duration of the current episode means the time between the patient's first experience of a clear change from normal life or mood and the time of the investigation. If the illness is recurrent, the current episode must have been preceeded by a clear illness-free interval of at least 3 months.

0: The episode has lasted less than 6 months.
1: The episode has lasted between 6 and 12 months.
2: The episode has lasted 1 year or more.

### Item R5 Character Neurosis

Character neurotic features may have emerged before the current episode, e.g. the patient's choice of spouse or life partner, (a peaceful or considerate companion rather than a dominating or self-assertive one) or style of life, because character neurotics avoid persons who provoke them. During the current episode the neurotic features may have manifested themselves in the way in which the patient presents his complaints, namely by striving for an emotional secondary gain. At the interview this striving can be observed in the patient's co-operation or in attention-demanding behaviour.

0: The patient has no sign of character neurosis.
1: It is uncertain whether the patient has a character neurosis.
2: The patient has shown clear signs of character neurosis.

## 5.3 Psychometric Description

*Type:* Diagnostic scale, which distinguishes between endogenous and reactive types in melancholia.

*Administration:* Observer scale. Semi-structured, goal-directed interview.

*Time axis:* The current episode of melancholia.

*Item selection:* Second generation scale. Developed on the basis of item analysis of the two Newcastle scales for depression [6].

*Number of items:* ten (five endogenous and five reactive items).

*Definition of items:* All items are defined according to operational criteria from 0 to 2.

*Psychometric validity:* The two dimensions in the scale fulfil the Rasch criteria for sufficient statistics, i.e. the total score is a sufficient measurement; no weighting as in the Newcastle scales is needed [6].

*Reliability:* Inter-observer reliability is adequate [6, 7].

*Comments:* The scale has recently been shown to be applicable and meaningful in general practice [8]. The most important item of the scale is "quality of depression" which covers the endogenous [9] or autonomous [10] separation between depressive illness and the emotional reaction to stress. When seen in the perspective of character neurosis [11] the depressive symptoms have no distinct quality because they have a deep personal association with the patient.

# References

1. Wing JK (1977) The limits of standardization. In: Rakoff WM, Stancer HC, Kedward HD (eds) Psychiatric diagnosis. Breunner-Mazel, New York
2. Hamilton M (1989) Frequency of symptoms in melancholia (depressive illness). Br J Psychiatry 154:201–206
3. American Psychiatric Association (1994) Diagnostic and statistical manual of mental disorders (DSM-IV), 4th edn. American Psychiatric Association, Washington DC
4. Kraepelin E (1921) Manic-depressive insanity and paranoia. Livingstone, Edinburgh
5. Freud S (1959) Mourning and melancholia. Collected papers (vol 4). Basic Books, New York
6. Bech P, Allerup P, Gram LF, Kragh-Sørensen P, Rafaelsen OJ, Reisby N, Vestergaard P and DUAG (1989) The Diagnostic Melancholia Scale (DMS). Dimensions of endogenous and reactive depression with relationship to the Newcastle Scales. J Affective Disord 14:161–170
7. Bech P (1993) Rating scales for psychopathology, health status and quality of life. Springer, Berlin Heidelberg New York
8. Fuglum E, Rosenberg C, Damsbo N, Stage K, Lauritzen L, Bech P and DUAG (1996) Screening and treating depressed patients. A comparison of two controlled citalopram trials across treatment settings: Hospitalized patients versus patients treated by their family doctors. Acta Psychiatr Scand (in press)
9. Roth M (1959) The phenomenology of depressive states. Canadian Psychiat Ass J 4 (Suppl):32–54
10. Gillepsie RD (1929) The clinical differentiation of types of depression. Guy's Hospital Reports 79:306–344
11. Partridge M (1949) Some reflections on the nature of affective disorders. J Ment Sci 95:795–825

# 6 The Zung Depression and Quality of Life Scales

## Contents

## 6.1 Introduction

In clinical research the issue of the administration of a scale in terms of observer ratings (scales administered by a skilled observer after an interview with the patient) versus self-rating scales (questionnaires to be completed by the patients themselves) has often been discussed. In mental disorders with reduced verbal capacity (e.g. dementia and mental handicaps) or reduced insight (e.g. schizophrenia, mania, and aggressiveness) the use of questionnaires is obviously very limited.

In the area of clinical depression observer scales such as the HAM-D and self-rating scales like the Beck Depression Inventory (BDI) [1] have most frequently been used. A meta-analysis has shown that in the acute therapy of depression the HAM-D is superior to BDI in discriminating between treatments. However, HAM-D and BDI cover different components of depressive states [1]. The most direct comparison between observer scales and questionnaires has been performed using the Zung depression scale, because this scale has both an observer form and a self-rating form [2, 3]. Results with the Zung scales have indicated that patients with mild to moderate degrees of depression, anxiety and subjective distress can communicate their discomfort and distress reliably. Whereas the BDI is a disease-dependent scale (i.e. a scale based on a specific theory of depression to be used in the subtypes of depressive illness for which cognitive therapy is indicated) the Zung Self Rating Depression Scale (Zung-SDS) is based on the affect balance scale, i.e. half of the items are positively worded (positive well-being) and the other half of items are negatively worded (negative well-being). This construction is also used in another self-rating scale, the Psychological General Well-Being Schedule [1]. The concept of health related quality of life refers to the patient's own perception of his or her problems during treatment. World Health Organization has recently published a well-being scale based on the Zung scales [4].

In this chapter the Zung Self Rating Depression Scale (Zung-SDS) has been included, as has the Zung Depression Scale (observer form), which, however, has been modified to measure major depression (Zung-MD), i.e. with reference to DSM-IV.

To cover quality of life scales the WHO (TEN) Well-Being Index (with reference to the Zung scales) has been included. Finally the PCASEE Scale, based on the DSM-IV multi-axial system, [1] has been included.

## 6.2 The Zung Self-Rating Depression Scale (ZUNG-SDS)

Please circle a number on each of the following statements to indicate how often you feel each of them has applied to you in the last week.

|  | None of the time | | | All of the time |
|---|---|---|---|---|
| 1. I feel down-hearted and sad | 1 | 2 | 3 | 4 |
| 2. Morning is when I feel best | 4 | 3 | 2 | 1 |
| 3. I have crying spells or feel like it | 1 | 2 | 3 | 4 |
| 4. I have trouble sleeping through the night | 1 | 2 | 3 | 4 |
| 5. I eat as much as I used to | 4 | 3 | 2 | 1 |
| 6. I enjoy looking at, talking to, and being with attractive women/men | 4 | 3 | 2 | 1 |
| 7. I notice that I am losing weight | 1 | 2 | 3 | 4 |
| 8. I have trouble with constipation | 1 | 2 | 3 | 4 |
| 9. My heart beats faster than usual | 1 | 2 | 3 | 4 |
| 10. I get tired for no reason | 1 | 2 | 3 | 4 |
| 11. My mind is as clear as it used to be | 4 | 3 | 2 | 1 |
| 12. I find it easy to do the things I used to do | 4 | 3 | 2 | 1 |
| 13. I am restless and can't keep still | 1 | 2 | 3 | 4 |
| 14. I feel hopeful about the future | 4 | 3 | 2 | 1 |
| 15. I am more irritable than usual | 1 | 2 | 3 | 4 |
| 16. I find it easy to make decisions | 4 | 3 | 2 | 1 |
| 17. I feel that I am useful and needed | 4 | 3 | 2 | 1 |
| 18. My life is pretty full | 4 | 3 | 2 | 1 |
| 19. I feel that others would be better off if I were dead | 1 | 2 | 3 | 4 |
| 20. I still enjoy the things I used to do | 4 | 3 | 2 | 1 |

The SDS criteria (standardization) for total score:

20–40: No depression                          48–55: Major depression
41–47: Less than major depression             56–80: More than major depression

## 6.3 The Zung Depression Scale for Major Depression with Reference to DSM-IV (Zung-MD)

| ICD-10 | DSM-IV | Zung items with an example question | DSM-IV/ ICD-10 diagnosis  Absent = 0 Present = 1 | Severity  0–3 |
|---|---|---|---|---|
| A1 | 1 | Do you feel sad or depressed? | | |
| A2 | 2 | Have you lost interests in things? (daily activities, family, friends) | | |
| A3 | 6 | Do you get tired easily? | | |
| B1 | 7 | Do you feel useless and not wanted? | | |
| B2 | 7 | Do you blame yourself for things? | | |
| B3 | 9 | Have you had thoughts about doing away with yourself? | | |
| B4 | 8 | Have you difficulties in making decisions? | | |
| B5 | 5 | Do you feel slowed down when doing the things you usually do? | | |
| B5 | 5 | Do you find yourself restless and unable to sit still? | | |
| B6 | 4 | Do you have trouble sleeping through the night? | | |
| B7 | 3 | Have you lost appetite and/or any weight? | | |

For diagnostic use the absence or presence of the symptoms during the last 2 weeks is completed. For severity, 0 = none of the time, 3 = all of the time during the last week.

*The DSM-IV criteria for major depression*: At least five of the nine symptoms.

*ICD-10 criteria for minor depression*: At least two A and two B symptoms.
*ICD-10 criteria for moderate depression*: At least two A and four B symptoms.
*ICD-10 criteria for severe depression*: All three A and at least five B symptoms.

## 6.4 The WHO (TEN) Well-Being Questionaire

Please circle a number on each of the following statements to indicate how often you feel each of them has applied to you in the past week.

|  | All of the time | | | None of the time |
|---|---|---|---|---|
| 1. I feel downhearted and sad | 0 | 1 | 2 | 3 |
| 2. I feel calm and peaceful | 3 | 2 | 1 | 0 |
| 3. I feel energetic, active or vigorous | 3 | 2 | 1 | 0 |
| 4. I wake up feeling fresh and rested | 3 | 2 | 1 | 0 |
| 5. I am happy, satisfied, or pleased with my personal life | 3 | 2 | 1 | 0 |
| 6. I feel well adjusted to my life situation | 3 | 2 | 1 | 0 |
| 7. I live the kind of life I want | 3 | 2 | 1 | 0 |
| 8. I feel eager to tackle my daily tasks or make new decisions | 3 | 2 | 1 | 0 |
| 9. I feel I can easily handle or cope with any serious problem or major change in my life | 3 | 2 | 1 | 0 |
| 10. My daily life is full of things that interest to me | 3 | 2 | 1 | 0 |

This version of the WHO (Ten) Well-Being Questionnaire is the European (British) adaptation of the American English Zung phrases. From 1996 it is the official WHO version placed in the European quarter, Copenhagen, Denmark.

## 6.5 The PCASEE Scale for Measuring Quality of Life

Below is a list of problems for complaints that people sometimes have. They are arranged so that there are five statements in each group. Please read each statement carefully. After you have done so, please fill in one of the boxes to the right that best describes how much that problem has bothered or distressed you during the past weeks including today.

| Group P Physical Problems | Group C Cognitive Problems | Group A Affective Problems | Group S Social Dysfunction | Group E Economic Problems | Group E Ego Problems |
|---|---|---|---|---|---|
| I sleep — badly □□□□□□ well | I concentrate — badly □□□□□□ well | I am anxious — severely □□□□□□ no | For my work I get — no appreciation □□□□□□ much appreciation | I am worried about money — definitely □□□□□□ no | My self-confidence is — poor □□□□□□ good |
| I feel physically — unwell □□□□□□ well | My memory is — poor □□□□□□ good | I want to get away from it al — definitely □□□□□□ no | I am doing household work — poorly □□□□□□ well | I am able to make ends meet — poorly □□□□□□ well | I feel sexually — unattractive □□□□□□ attractive |
| My appetite is — poor □□□□□□ good | I am able to make decisions — poorly □□□□□□ well | I feel comfortable with myself — no □□□□□□ definitely | I perform any work — poorly □□□□□□ well | I am able to buy what I want — no □□□□□□ definitely | My feelings are hurt — too easily □□□□□□ not easily |
| I experience physical pain — severe □□□□□□ no | I feel in control of life — badly □□□□□□ well | I am sad — severely □□□□□□ no | My interest in my daily activities is — poor □□□□□□ good | I am able to buy what I need — no □□□□□□ definitely | I can forgive myself — not easily □□□□□□ easily |
| My energy is — lacking □□□□□□ full | My thinking is — unclear □□□□□□ clear | I am irritable — severely □□□□□□ no | My social life is — poor □□□□□□ good | I need financial assistance — definitely □□□□□□ no | What I want from life is — unclear □□□□□□ clear |

## 6.6 Psychometric Description
### of the Zung Self-Rating Depression Scale (ZUNG-SDS)

*Type:* Symptom scale.

*Subject area:* Depression: severity of the illness and measuring change in depressive states during treatment.

*Administration:* Self-administered by the patient.

*Item selection:* First generation scale based on the same domain of depressive symptomatology as the HAM-D scale. A coefficient between the two scales of 0.80 has been found [11].

*Number of items:* 20.

*Definition of items:* The quantifier is not intensity of symptoms but frequency, which also is the approach used in self-rating scales for quality of life.

*Comments:* The scale is the most frequently used self-rating scale in the pharmacotherapy of depression. The 4 factors identified by Zung [2] are with the item numbers in brackets: 1 Mood symptoms (1, 3); 2 Somatic symptoms (2, 4, 5, 6, 7, 8, 9, 10); 3 Psychomotor symptoms (12, 13); and 4 Cognitive symptoms (11, 14, 15, 16, 17, 18, 19, 20). The first well-being index was identified in 1975 [12].

## 6.7 Psychometric Description of the Health-Related Quality
### of Life Scales

The Zung Depression Scale is originally a 20 item questionnaire (Sect. 6.2). The version in Sect. 6.3 is tailored to DSM-IV and ICD-10. However, whereas DSM-IV and ICD-10 define depression as a syndrome of symptoms that should has been constantly present during the last 2 weeks, the Zung items are measured in frequency. The Zung scale is included here for the measurement of the outcome of treatment, as are the other quality of life scales.

The WHO scale was constructed by Bradley [5–7] on similar lines to the Zung scales [2]. The total of 28 items in the scale were psychometrically analysed by Bech et al. [4], resulting in the ten item version (Sect. 6.4). The construct validity of the scale in terms of homogeneity coefficients has been found adequate (Cronbach alpha = 0.85, Loevinger = 0.40). This analysis was made on 358 patients with diabetes selected in different European centres.

These psychometric results with the WHO (Ten) Well-Being Scale have recently been confirmed in a cross-national study in psychiatric settings (Report on a WHO consensus meeting, November 1996).

The PCASEE scale was constructed by Bech [1] on the basis of results with the Smith Kline Beecham Quality of Life Scale (SBQOL) [8]. The scale consists of 6×5 items (see Sect. 6.5), i.e. 30 items. Each item is scored from 0

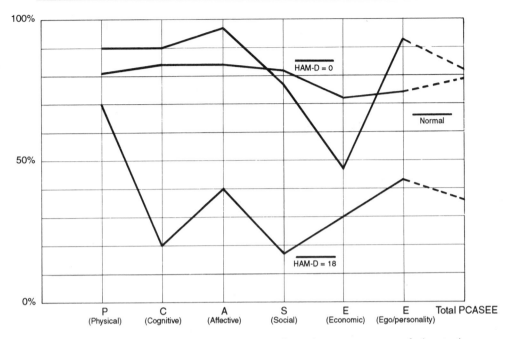

**Fig. 2.** The PCASEE profiles and total scores transformed to a percentage scale (see text). Higher scores mean better well-being

(e.g. unwell or poor) to 5 (e.g. well or good). Thus, higher scores indicate better well-being analogue to the Psychological General Well-Being Schedule [1]. Each of the six PCASEE components (P = physical indicators; C = cognitive indicators; A = affective indicators; S = social indicators; E = economic-social indicators; and E = ego or personality indicators) are the scored (analogue to the SF-36 [1] from 0 to 100). Figure 2 shows a patient under long-term, pro-phylactic treatment for depression, who dropped from 0 to 18 on the HAM-D. For comparison a sample of normal students is shown. The impact of depres-sion (HAM-D = 18) is easily seen on Figure 2, both as a profile score and as total score (higher scores mean better well-being). It has recently been shown [9] that the PCASEE and to a less extent the Psychological General Well-Being Schedule [1, 10] were capable of predicting recurrences of major depressive episodes.

## References

1. Bech P (1993) Rating scales for psychopathology, health status and quality of life. A compendium on documentation in accordance with the DSM-III-R and WHO systems. Springer, Berlin Heidelberg New York.
2. Zung WWK (1965) A self-rating depression scale. Arch Gen Psychiatry 12:63–70

3. Tegeler J, Klieser E, Heinrich K (1990) Double-blind study of the therapeutic efficacy and tolerability of amitriptylinoxide in comparison with amitriptyline. Pharmaco-psychiatry 23:45–49
4. Bech P, Staehr Johansen K, Gudex C (1996) The WHO (Ten) Well-Being Index: Validation in Diabetes. Psychotherapy and Psychosomatics (in press)
5. Meadows K, Bradley C (1990) Report to World Health Organization. European quarter, Copenhagen
6. Bradley C (ed) (1994) Handbook of psychology and diabetes: a guide to psychological measurement in diabetes research and practice. Harwood, London
7. Warr PB, Banks MH, Ullah P (1985) The experience of unemployment among black and white urban teenagers. Br J Psychol 76:75–87
8. Dunbar GC, Stoker MJ, Hodges TCP, Beaumont G (1992) The development of SBQOL: an unique scale for measuring the quality of life. Br J Med Econ 2:65–74
9. Thunedborg K, Black C, Bech P (1995) Beyond the Hamilton Depression Scale scores in manic- melancholic patients in long term relapse-prevention: a quality of life approach. Psychother and Psychosom 64:131–140
10. Dupuy HJ (1984) The psychological general well-being (PGWB) index: an assessment of quality of life in clinical trials of cardiovascular therapies. In: Wenger NK, Mattson ME, Furberg CD, Elison J (eds) Le Jacq, New York, pp 184–188
11. Biggs JT, Wylie CT, Ziegler V (1978) Validity of the Zung Self-rating Depression Scale. Brit J Psychiat 132:381–385
12. Blumenthal MD (1975) Measuring depression symptomatology in a general population. Arch Gen Psychiatry 32:971–978

# Appendix 1.
# The Hamilton Depression Scale (HAM-D) Combined with the Melancholia Scale (MES) and the Montgomery Åsberg Scale (MADRS)

**Contents**

## 1.1 Introduction

This updated version of the Bech, Hamilton, Newcastle and Zung scales is an attempt to revise well-known scales instead of introducing new ones. However, many new depression scales have been developed during the last decades, among them the Montgomery Åsberg Scale [1], the Widlöcher Retardation Scale and the Cornell Dysthymia Scale [2]. Of these scales the Montgomery Åsberg Scale (MADRS) has been most frequently used as an index of depressive states in psychopharmacology. In Sect. 1.2 the scoring sheet for the combined HAM-D/MES and the corresponding MADRS items is given. Among the global scales which should be mentioned in this context are the Clinical Global Impression Scale (CGI) and the Visual Analogue Scale (VAS) [3]. The CGI is scored: 1 = not at all depressed, 2 = doubtfully depressed, 3 = mildly depressed, 4 = moderately depressed, 5 = markedly depressed, 6 = severely depressed, and 7 = among the most extremely depressed patients. The updated version of the clinical Global Impression Scale ranging from 0 to 10 is shown in Table 1. The CGI is often referred to as a Graphical Rating Scale [4]. In comparison, the VAS is a 10 cm horizontal line with "no depression" at the left end and "among the most extremely depressed patients" at the right end.

The primary outcome measure in trials with antidepressants is a 50 percent reduction in the pretreatment (baseline) HAM-D score [5]. When comparing HAM-D and MADRS in a meta-analysis of randomized clinical trials with citalopram [6] a 50 percent reduction in the pretreatment scores was most appropriate. This outcome criterion equals "very much" plus "much" improved according to the Clinical Global Improvement Scale [5, 6].

## 1.2 Scoring Sheet

Scoring sheet for the Melancholia Scale (MES) integrated with the Hamilton Depression Scale (HAM-D) with the corresponding Montgomery Åsberg (MADRS) items

| DSM-IV | No. | Item | HAM-D | MES | MADRS | ICD-10 |
|--------|-----|------|-------|-----|-------|--------|
| 1 | 1 | Depressed mood | ☐ | ☐ | ☐a ☐b | A1 |
| 7 | 2 | Low self-esteem, guilt | ☐ | ☐ | ☐ | B1, B2 |
| 9 | 3 | Sucidical thoughts | ☐ | ☐ | ☐ | B3 |
| 4 | 4 | Insomnia: initial | ☐ | | | B6 |
| 4 | 5 | Insomnia: middle | ☐ | | | B6 |
| 4 | 6 | Insomnia: late | ☐ | | | B6 |
| 2 | 7 | Social life activities and interests | ☐ | ☐ | ☐ | A2 |
| 5 | 8 | Psychomotor retardation: general | ☐ | | | B5 |
| 5 | 9 | Psychomotor agitation | ☐ | | | B5 |
| | 10 | Anxiety: psychic | ☐ | ☐ | ☐ | |
| | 11 | Anxiety: somatic | ☐ | | | |
| 3 | 12 | Gastrointestinal symptoms | ☐ | | ☐ | B7 |
| 6 | 13 | Somatic symptoms: general | ☐ | | | A3 |
| | 14 | Sexual disturbances | ☐ | | | |
| | 15 | Hypochondriasis (somatization) | ☐ | | | |
| | 16 | Insight | ☐ | | | |
| 3 | 17 | Weight loss | ☐ | | | B7 |
| 4 | 18 | Insomnia: general | | ☐ | ☐ | B6 |
| 5 | 19 | Decreased motor activity | | ☐ | | B5 |
| 5 | 20 | Decreased verbal activity | | ☐ | | B5 |
| 8 | 21 | Concentration difficulties | | ☐ | ☐ | B4 |
| 2 | 22 | Introversion | | ☐ | ☐ | A2 |
| 6 | 23 | Tiredness | | ☐ | | A3 |
| | | Total | HAM-D ☐☐ | MES ☐☐ | MADRS ☐☐ | |

*The DSM-IV criteria for major depression*: Each of the nine DSM-IV items has a score of 1 if the corresponding HAM-D/MES item has a positive score. Major depression is then defined by a score of 1 on at least five of the nine items.

*The ICD-10 criteria for minor depression*: A score of 1 or more on two of the three A items and on two of the seven B items.

*ICD-10 criteria for moderate depression*: A score of 1 or more on the two of the three A items and on four of the seven B items.

*ICD-10 criteria for severe depression*: A score of 1 or more on all three A items and on five of the seven B items.

# 1.3 Item Definitions for the HAM-D MES with Corresponding MADRS Items

## HAM-D/MES

### MADRS

---

1. Depressed mood

Covers verbal and non-verbal communication of sadness, despair, despondency, helplessness and hopelessness.
0: Not present.
1: Very mild tendencies to lowered spirits.
2: The patient is more clearly concerned by unpleasant experiences although he or she still lacks feelings of hopelessness.
3: Moderately to markedly depressed. Some hopelessness and/or clear non-verbal signs of depression.
4: Severe degree of lowered mood. Pronounced hopelessness.

---

1a. Apparent sadness

Representing despondency, gloom and despair (more than just ordinary transient low spirits), reflected in speech, facial expression, and posture. Rate by depth and inability to brighten up.
0: No sadness.
2: Looks dispirited but does brighten up without difficulty.
4: Appears sad and unhappy most of the time.
6: Looks miserable all the time. Extremely despondent

---

1b. Reported sadness

Representing reports of depressed mood, regardless of whether it is reflected in appearance or not. Includes low spirits, despondency or the feeling of being beyond help and without hope.
0: Occasional sadness in keeping with the circumstances.
2: Sad or low but brightens up without difficulty.
4: Pervasive feelings of sadness or gloominess. The mood is still influenced by external circumstances.
6: Continuous or unvarying sadness, misery or despondency.

---

2. Low self-esteem and Guilt

Covers negative self-esteem, self-depreciation or guilt feelings.
0: Not present.
1: Concerned with the fact of being a burden to the family, friends or colleagues due to reduced interests, introversion, low capacity or loss of self-esteem/self- confidence.
2: Self-depreciation or guilt feelings are clearly present because the patient is concerned with incidents (minor omissions or failures) in the past prior to the current episode of depression.
3: Feels that current depression is a punishment but can still see intellectually that this view is unfounded.
4: Guilt feelings have become paranoid ideas.

---

2. Pessimistic thoughts

Representing thoughts of guilt, inferiority, self-reproach, sinfulness, remorse and ruin.
0: No pessimistic thoughts.
2: Fluctuating ideas of failure, self-reproach or self- depreciation.
4: Persistent self-accusations, or definite but still rational ideas of guilt or sin. Increasingly pessimistic about the future.
6: Delusions of ruin, remorse or irredeemable sin. Self- accusations which are absurd and unshakable.

## HAM-D/MES                                    MADRS

3. Suicidal thoughts

Covers suicidal tendencies or plans. Is rated in degrees of probability of acting.
0: Not present.
1: The patient feels that life is not worthwhile, but expresses no wish to die.
2: The patient wishes to die but has no plans for taking his/her own life.
3: Probably has plans to hurt himself/herself.
4: Definitely has plans to kill himself/herself

3. Suicidal thoughts

Representing the feeling that life is not worth living, that a natural death would be welcome, suicidal thoughts, and preparations for suicide. Suicide attempts should not in themselves influence the rating.
0: Enjoys life or takes it as it comes.
2: Weary of life. Only fleeting suicidal thoughts.
4: Probably better off dead. Suicidal thoughts are common, and suicide is considered as a possible solution, but without specific plans or intenstion.
6: Explicit plans for suicide when there is an opportunity. Active preparations for suicide.

4., 5., 6., 18.

The administration of sedatives or hypnotic drugs should not in themselves influence rating

4. Initial insomnia

0: Not present
1: At least 1 of the last 3 nights the patient lay in bed for more than 30 min before falling asleep.
: Each of the 3 nights the patient lay in bed for more than 30 min before falling asleep.

5. Middle insomnia

Wakes up one or more times between midnight and 5 a.m.
0: Not present.
1: Once or twice during the last 3 nights.
2: At least once every night.

6. Late insomnia

Wakes up before planned.
0: Not present.
1: Less than 1 hour too early (and may fall asleep again).
2: Constantly, or more than 1 hour too early.

18. General insomnia

0: Usual sleep duration.
1: Duration of sleep slightly reduced.
2: Duration of sleep clearly reduced but still moderate, i.e. still less than an 50% reduction.
3: Duration of sleep markedly reduced.
4: Duration of sleep extremely reduced, e.g. as if not been sleeping at all

18. Reduced sleep

Representing the experience of reduced duration or depth of sleep compared to the subject's own normal pattern when well.
0: Sleeps as normal.
2: Slight difficulty dropping off to sleep or slightly reduced, light or fitful sleep.
4: Sleep reduced or broken by at least 2 hours.
6: Less than 2 hours sleep.

## HAM-D/MES

**7. Social life activities and interests**

Should be rated in degree of efficiency in social life functioning.

0: No difficulties; feels time useful.
1: Mild insufficiencies in social life activities; patient feels that he/she does not do enough with social life activities.
2: Clear little interest or pleasure in doing things but still only moderate insufficiencies in the patient's day-to-day activities.
3: Difficulties in performing even daily routine activities, which are carried out with great effort.
4: Often needs help in performing self care activities (unable to function independently).

**8. Psychomotor retardation, general**

0: Not present.
1: Conversational speed scarcely or slightly reduced and facial expression scarcely or slightly stiffened (retarded).
2: Conversational speed clearly reduced, with intermissions; reduced gestures and slow pace.
3: The interview is clearly prolonged due to long breaks and brief answers; all movements are very slow.
4: The interview cannot be completed; retardation approaches (and includes) stupor.

**9. Psychomotor agitation**

0: Not present.
1: Doubtful or slight agitation, for example, tendency to changing position in chair or at times scratching his head.
2: Fidgeting; wringing hands, clearly changing position in chair now and again; clearly, but still moderately restless in ward, with some pacing.
3: Patient cannot stay in chair during interview (and/or much pacing in ward).
4: Interview must be conducted "on the run". Almost continuous pacing; pulling off clothes, tearing his hair.

## MADRS

**7. Lassitude**

Representing difficulty in getting started or slowness in initiating and performing everyday activities.

0: Hardly any difficulty in getting started. No sluggishness.
2: Difficulties in starting activities.
4: Difficulties in starting simple routine activities which are carried out with effort.
6: Complete lassitude. Unable to do anything without help.

## HAM-D/MES

10. Anxiety: psychic

0: Not present.
1: Very mild tendencies to tenseness, worry, fear or apprehension.
2: The patient is more clearly in a state of anxiety, apprehension or insecurity, which, however, he or she is still able to control.
3: The anxiety or apprehension is at times more difficult to control. For example, patient at the edge of panic.
4: Extreme degree of anxiety, interfering greatly with patient's daily life.

11. Anxiety: somatic

0: The patient is neither more nor less prone than usual to experience the somatic concomitants of psychic anxety states.
1: The patient occasionally experiences slight manifestations, such as abdominal symptoms, sweating or trembling; however, the description is vague and doubtful.
2: The patient from time to time experiences abdominal symptoms, sweating, trembling, etc. Symptoms and signs are clearly described but are not marked or incapacitating, i.e. still without influence on the patient's daily life.
3: Physiological concomitants of anxious states are marked and sometimes very worrying. They interfere occasionally with the patient's daily life.
4: Physiological concomitants of anxious states are numerous, persistent and often incapacitating. They interfere markedly with the patient's daily life.

## MADRS

10. Inner tension

Representing feelings of ill-defined discomfort, edginess, inner turmoil, mental tension mounting to either panic, dread or anguish. Rate according to intensity, frequency, duration and the extent of reassurance called for.
0: Placid. Only fleeting inner tension.
2: Occasional feelings of edginess and ill-defined discomfort.
4: Continuous feelings of inner tension or intermittent panic which the patient can only master with some difficulty.
6: Unrelenting dread or anguish. Overwhelming panic.

## HAM-D/MES                                    ## MADRS

12. Gastrointestinal symptoms (appetite)

0: No gastrointestinal complaints (or symptoms unchanged from before onset of depression).
1: Food intake is about normal, but without relish (all dishes taste alike and/or cigarettes are without flavour).
2: Food intake is reduced; the patient must often be urged to eat.

12. Reduced appetite

Representing the feeling of a loss of appetite compared with when well. Rate by loss of desire for food or the need to force oneself to eat.
0: Normal or increased appetite.
2: Slightly reduced appetite.
4: No appetite. Food is tasteless.
6: Needs persuasion to eat at all.

17. Weight loss

A: At first rating
0: No weight loss.
1: Weight loss of 1–2.5 kg.
2: Weight loss of 3 kg or more.

B: At weekly interviews
0: No weight loss.
1: Weight loss of 0.5 kg per week.
2: Weight loss of 1 kg or more per week.

## HAM-D/MES

13. Somatic symptoms: general

0: The patient is neither more nor less tired or troubled by bodily discomfort than usual.
1: Doubtful or very vague feelings of muscular fatigue or other somatic discomfort.
2: The patient is clearly or constantly tired and exhausted, and/or troubled by bodily discomforts (e.g. muscular headache).

14. Sexual disturbances

0: No disturbances.
1: Doubtful or mild reduction in sexual interest and enjoyment.
2: Clear loss of sexual appetite. Often functional impotence in men and lack of arousal or plain disgust in women.

15. Hypochondriasis (somatization)

0: The patient pays no more interest than usual to the slight bodily sensations of everyday life.
1: Slightly more occupied than usual with bodily symptoms and functions.
2: The patient is quite worried about his physical health. He/she expresses thoughts of organic disease, with a tendency to somatize the clinical presentation.
3: The patient is convinced he/she is suffering from a physical illness which can explain all his/her symptoms (brain tumour, abdominal cancer, etc.), but he/she can briefly be reassured that this is not the case.
4: The preoccupation with bodily dysfunction has clearly reached paranoid dimensions. The hypochondriac delusions often have a nihilistic quality or guilt associations: to be rotting inside; insects eating the tissues; bowels blocked and withering away; other patients are being infected by the patient's bad odour or his/her syphilis. Counter-argumentation is without effect.

**HAM-D/MES**

16. Insight

0: The patient agrees that he/she has depressive symptoms or a similar nervous illness.
1: The patient agrees that he/she is depressed but feels this to be secondary to conditions unrelated to the illness such as malnutrition, climate, or overwork.
2: The patient denies being ill at all. Delusional patients are by definition without insight. Enquiries should therefore be directed to the patient's attitude to his symptoms of guilt (item 2) or hypochondriasis (item 15), but other delusional symptoms should also be considered.

19. Decreased motor activity

0: Not present.
1: Very mild tendencies to decreased motor activity, for example, facial expression slightly retarded.
2: Moderately reduced motor activity, e.g. facial expression more clearly rigid, the head bent forward, looking down, reduced gestures.
3: Markedly reduced motor activity, e.g. all movements slow.
4: Severely reduced motor activity, approaching stupor.

20. Decreased verbal activity

0: Not present.
1: Very mild tendencies to reduced verbal formulation activity.
2: More pronounced inertia in conversation, for example, a tendency to longer intermissions.
3: Interview is clearly coloured by brief responses or long pauses.
4: Interview is clearly prolonged due to decreased verbal formulation activity.

## HAM-D/MES

### 21. Concentration difficulties

Covers difficulties in concentration, in decisions about everyday matters.

0: Not present.
1: Very mild tendencies to concentration disturbances or problems in decision making.
2: Even with a major effort patient finds it difficult to concentrate occasionally.
3: Difficulties in concentration even in things that usually need no effort (reading a newspaper, watching television programme).
4: When it is clear that the patient is also showing difficulties in concentration during interview.

### 22. Introversion

Covers the reduced emotional contact with other human beings.

0: Not present.
1: Very mild tendencies to emotional indifference in relation to social surroundings (colleagues).
2: The patient is more clearly emotionally introverted in relation to colleagues or other people but still glad to be with friends or family.
3: Moderately to markedly introverted, i.e. less need or ability to feel warmth to friends or family.
4: The patient feels isolated or emotionally indifferent even to near friends or family.

### 23. Tiredness

0: Not present.
1: Very mild feelings of tiredness.
2: The patient is more clearly in a state of tiredness and weakness, but these symptoms are still without influence on the patient's daily life.
3: Marked feelings of tiredness which interfere occasionally with the patient's daily life.
4: Extreme feelings of tiredness interfering more constantly with the patient's daily life.

## MADRS

### 21. Concentration difficulties

Representing difficulties in collecting one's thoughts mounting to an incapacitating lack of concentration. Rate according to intensity, frequency, and degree of incapacity produced.

0: No difficulties in concentrating.
2: Occasional difficulties in collecting one's thoughts.
4: Difficulties in concentrating and sustaining thought which reduced ability to read or hold a conversation.
6: Unable to read or converse without great difficulty.

### 22. Inability to feel

Representing the subjective experience of reduced interest in the surroundings, or activities that normally give pleasure. The ability to react with adequate emotion to circumstances or people is reduced.

0: Normal interest in the surroundings and in other people.
2: Reduced ability to enjoy usual interests.
4: Loss of interest in the surroundings. Loss of feelings for friends and acquaintances.
6: The experience of being emotionally paralysed, inability to feel anger, grief or pleasure and a complete or even painful failure to feel for close relatives and friends.

## 1.4 HAM-D/MES Criteria for Major Depression

The standardization of HAM-D (17 item total score) in relationship to major depression is:

| HAM-D scores | Categories |
|---|---|
| 0–7 | No depression |
| 8–12 | Minor depression |
| 13–17 | Less than major depression |
| 18–29 | Major depression |
| 30–52 | More than major depression |

## 1.5 HAM-D/MES Factors or Indexes

The most frequently used factors are:

(1) The Melancholia (depression) index:
    HAM-D items 1, 2, 7, 8, 10, 13

(2) The anxiety index:
    HAM-D items 9, 10, 11

(3) The sleep index:
    HAM-D items 4, 5, 6

## References

1. Montgomery SA, Åsberg M (1979) A new depression scale to be sensitive to change. Br J Psychiatry 134:382–389
2. Widlöcher DJ (1983) Psychomotor retardation: clinical, theoretical, and psychometric aspects. Psychiatr Clin North Am 6:27–40
3. Bech P (1993) Rating scales for psychopathology, health status and quality of life. Springer, Berlin Heidelberg New York.
4. Hersen M, Bellack AS (1988) Dictionary of behavioral assessment techniques. Pergamon Press, New York, p 490.
5. Depression Guideline Panel (1993) Depression in primary care, 2: Treatment of major depression. US Department of Health and Human Services. (AHCPR publication 93-0551), Rockville, Maryland
6. Bech P (1989) Clinical properties of citalopramin comparison with other antidepressants: A quantitative meta-analysis. In: Montgomery SA (ed) Citalopram Excerpta Medica, Amsterdam, pp 56–68
7. Paykal ES (1990) Use of the Hamilton Depression Scale in general practice. In: Bech P, Coppen A (eds) The Hamilton Scales. Springer, Berlin Heidelberg New York, pp 40–77

# Appendix 2.
# The Melancholia Scale for Brief and Major Depression (MES/BMD)

**Contents**

## 2.1 Scoring Sheet with Standardizations and Item Definitions

| No. | Item<br>The scale covers the last 14 days | Score | |
|---|---|---|---|
| | | Frequency<br>$(0-4)$ | Intensity<br>$(0-4)$ |
| 1 | Interests<br>(lost interest in ordinary day-to-day activities, difficulties getting going) | | |
| 2 | Lowered mood<br>(lowering of spirits, crying spells, hopelessness) | | |
| 3 | Sleep disturbances<br>(falling asleep, restless sleep, early waking) | | |
| 4 | Anxiety or inner unrest<br>(difficulties in relaxing, feeling fearful, been worrying too much, scared, insecure) | | |
| 5 | Emotional introversion<br>(felt lonely, avoid contact with friends or family, avoid meetings or other arrangements) | | |
| 6 | Concentration disturbances<br>(trouble keeping your mind on what you are doing, e.g. when reading a book or watching TV) | | |
| 7 | Tiredness<br>(everything an effort, easily tired) | | |
| 8 | Low self-esteem, guilt feelings<br>(not so good as others blaming yourself for things) | | |
| 9 | Reduced verbal activity or performance<br>(talking less than usual, quiet, long intervals in conversation) | | |
| 10 | Suicidal thoughts<br>(life seems pointless, thoughts of ending your life) | | |
| 11 | Reduced motor activity<br>(movements slow, felt you look older) | | |
| | | Typical frequency score<br>☐ | Total<br>☐☐ |

| | |
|---|---|
| *Frequency* is scored as follows: | 0 = not present; 1 = rarely (1 day or less); 2 = some of the time (2 – 4 days); 3 = often (5 – 8 days); 4 = constantly (9 or more days) |
| *Intensity* is scored as follows: | 0 = not present; 1 = very mild; 2 = mild to moderate; 3 = moderate to marked; 4 = marked to extreme |
| *Brief Depression Score*: | The typical frequency item score of 2 or less |
| *Major Depression Score*: | The intensity total score of 15 or more |
| *Less than major Depression Score*: | The intensity total score of 10 to 14 |

## 2.2 Psychometric Description

*Type:* Symptom scale.

*Subject area:* Depression: severity and frequency of symptoms.

*Administration:* Observer scale; semi-structured, goal-directed interview.

*Time axis:* The previous 14 days.

*Item selection:* The eleven items are identical with the MES.

*Number of items:* 11.

*Definition of items:* The item definitions are based on the self-rating version of MES [1]. However, whereas the MES only measures the intensity of symptoms (because major depression according to DSM-IV or ICD-10 requires that the symptoms have been present nearly every day during the last 14 days), the MES/BMD also measure frequency (according to ICD-10 a brief depression typically lasts 2 – 3 days).

*Psychometric validity:* The content validity for intensity scores of MES/BMD equals in symptom profile both DSM-IV and ICD-10. The content validity for frequency equals one of the most used screening scales, the CES-D [2]. The scale was developed [3] from an ongoing study in patients with Parkinson's disease (PD). Patients suffering from PD have a more fluctuating symptomatology than patients with post-stroke depression. In the latter category of patients the MES has been found to have a better discriminatory validity than the HAM-D [4]. The MES/BMD has the ability to capture the fluctuating symptomatology which often swings between "brief recurrent depression" and "major depression" [3].

*Comments:* Studies with the MES/BMD are in progress both in PD and in depression in the elderly. Because the interview version seems applicable also in patients with decreased verbal capacity, the scale is recommended for use in dementia and mental handicap.

# References

1. Bech P (1993) Rating scales for psychopathology, health status, and quality of life. A compendium on documentation in accordance with the DSM-III-R and WHO systems. Springer, Berlin Heidelberg New York
2. Radloff LS (1977) The CES-D scale. A self-report depression scale for research in the general population. Appl Psychol Measurement 1:385–401
3. Bech P (1993) Depressive syndrome in Parkinson's disease: clinical manifestations. In: Wolters EC, Scheltens P (eds) Mental dysfunction in Parkinson's disease. Vrije Universiteit Press Amsterdam, pp 315–324
4. Lauritzen L, Bjerg Bendsen B, Vilmar T, Bjerg Bendsen E, Lunde M, Bech P (1994) Post-stroke depression: combined treatment with imipramine or desipramine and mianserin. A controlled clinical study. Psychopharmacology (Berl) 114:119–122

# Appendix 3.
# Major Depression Rating Based on the HAM-D and MES (MDS) Scales

**Contents**

## 3.1 Introduction

The term "major depression" is used as the main indication for antidepressants in many countries outside North America, i.e. in countries where ICD-10 rather than DSM-IV is the official diagnostic system. Especially in the setting of general practice where most of the antidepressants are prescribed, it is important to specify the nine symptoms constituting major depression in more detail. With this background the scoring sheet for "Major depression rating based on HAM-D/MES" has been included here with the corresponding item definitions. The theoretical score range is up to 36. However, a score profile with a score of at least 2 on five of the nine items is the equivalent of DSM-IV major depression, i.e. a total score of 10. The rating of major depression provides a better way to express degrees of remission during treatment than the number of symptoms. In other words the major depression rating based on HAM-D/MES (MDS) is an outcome measure. The scale has been validated in different clinical settings (psychiatric hospitals, private psychiatric practice, and general practice) when compared to the HAM-D and MES [1]. The results showed a high internal validity (better than HAM-D and equal to MES) in terms of Loevinger coefficients of homogeneity and factor analysis (one general factor only). The inter-observer reliability was equal to HAM-D and MES (0.83 in terms of intra-class correlation). In another study [2] it has been shown that the items of the Major Depression Rating Scale are not influenced by age or sex of the patients. Preliminary analysis of the Major Depression Scale has shown that a total score of 12 equals major depression on HAM-D (i.e. a total score on HAM-D of 18) or MES (i.e. a total score on MES of 15).

A structured interview guide has been included the item definitions. The time frame has not been included because it differs from study to study. When screening for a diagnosis the last two weeks is the time frame. When reassessing the patient during a treatment period the last week or the last three days are most appropriate. The structured interview guide has been developed with reference to Williams [3], but with some modifications.

## 3.2 Scoring Sheet
## Major Depression Rating Scale (DSM-IV Version)

| ITEM | | Score |
|------|------|-------|
| 1. Depressed mood | (0−4) | |
| 2. Diminished interests in social activities | (0−4) | |
| 3. Decreased appetite and/or significant weight loss (sum of 3a and 3b) <br> 3a Decreased appetite (0−2) <br> 3b Weight loss (0−2) | (0−4) | |
| 4. Insomnia | (0−4) | |
| 5. Psychomotor retardation and/or agitation (highest score on 5a or 5b) <br> 5a Retardation (0−4) <br> 5b Agitation (0−4) | (0−4) | |
| 6. Fatigue or loss of energy | (0−4) | |
| 7. Feelings of worthlessness or guilt | (0−4) | |
| 8. Diminished ability to concentrate | (0−4) | |
| 9. Recurrent thoughts of death, suicidal ideas or plans | (0−4) | |
| TOTAL SCORE | (0−36) | |

## 3.3 Structure Interview Guide and Item Definitions

### General Remarks

The interview should assess the presence and intensity of the nine items over a minimum period of three days.

### 1 Depressed Mood

What's your mood been like? Have you been feeling sad or unhappy? Depressed at all? Hopeless?

> Covers verbal and non-verbal communication of sadness, despair, despondency, helplessness and hopelessness.
>
> 0: Not present.
> 1: Very mild tendencies to lowered spirits.
> 2: The patient is more clearly concerned by unpleasant experiences although he or she still lacks feelings of hopelessness.
> 3: Moderately to markedly depressed. Some hopelessness and/or clear non-verbal signs of depression.
> 4: Severe degree of lowered mood. Pronounced hopelessness.

## 2 Diminished Interests in Social Activities

Have you felt interested in doing the things you should do, or do you feel you have to push yourself to do them? Have you stopped doing anything you used to do?

---

Should be rated in degree of efficiency in social life functioning. Covers also motivation, i.e. lack of interest or pleasure in doing things.

0: No difficulties; feels time spent usefully.
1: Mild insufficiencies in social life activities; patient feels that he/she does not do enough with social life activities.
2: Clear (little interest or pleasure in doing things) but still only moderate insufficiencies in the patient's day-to-day activities.
3: Difficulties in performing even daily routine activities, which are carried out with great effort.
4: Often needs help in performing self care activities (unable to function independently).

---

## 3 Decreased Appetite and/or Significant Weight Loss

How has your appetite been? What about compared to your usual appetite? Have you had to force yourself to eat? Have other people had to urge you to eat?
Have you lost weight since this (depression) began?
If not sure: Do you think your clothes are any looser on you?

---

3a Decreased appetite

0: Not present.
1: Food intake is about or slightly less than normal; but without relish or tasteless.
2: Food intake is significantly reduced.

3b Weight loss

0: No weight loss.
1: Weight loss of 0.5 kg per week (or 1–2.5 kg in the current depressive episode).
2: Weight loss of 1 kg or more per week (or 3 kg or more in the current episode).

---

## 4 General Insomnia

How has your sleeping been? Have you had trouble staying asleep? How many hours have you slept on the last three nights in average.

---

0: Usual sleep duration.
1: Duration of sleep slightly reduced.
2: Duration of sleep clearly reduced but still moderate, i.e. still less than an 50% reduction.
3: Duration of sleep markedly reduced.
4: Duration of sleep extremely reduced, e.g., as if had not been sleeping at all.

## 5 Psychomotor Retardation and/or Agitation

Rating based on observations during interview.

5a Retardation

0: Not present.
1: Conversational speed doubtfully or slightly reduced and facial expression doubt-fully or slightly stiffened (retarded).
2: Conversational speed clearly reduced, with intermissions; reduced gestures and slow pace.
3: The interview is clearly prolonged due to long pauses and brief answers; all move-ments are very slow.
4: The interview cannot be completed; retardation approaches (and includes) stupor.

5b Agitation

0: Not present.
1: Doubtful or slight agitation, e. g., tendency to change position in chair or at times scratch his head.
2: Fidgeting; wringing hands, clearly changing position in chair now and again; clearly, but still moderately restless in ward, with some pacing.
3: Patient cannot stay in chair during interview (and/or much pacing in ward).
4: Interview must be conducted "on the run". Almost continuous pacing; pulling off clothes, tearing his hair.

## 6 Fatigue or Loss of Energy

How has your energy been? Have you been tired? Have you had any trouble getting started at things?

0: Not present.
1: Very mild feelings of tiredness.
2: The patient is more clearly in a state of tiredness and weakness, but these symp-toms are still without influence on the patient's daily life.
3: Marked feelings of tiredness which interfere occasionally with the patient's daily life.
4: Extreme feelings of tiredness interfering more constantly with the patient's daily life.

## 7 Feelings of Worthlessness or Guilt

Have you been especially critical of yourself or been feeling guilty? How about blaming yourself for things? Have you felt that you're a failure in some way?

> Covers negative self-esteem, self-depreciation or guilt feelings.
>
> 0: Not present.
> 1: Concerned with the fact of being a burden to the family, friends or colleagues due to reduced interests, introversion, low capacity or loss of self-esteem/self-confidence.
> 2: Self-depreciation or guilt feelings are clearly present because the patient is concerned with incidents (minor omissions or failures) in the past prior to the current episode of depression.
> 3: Feels that current depression is a punishment but can still see intellectually that this view is unfounded.
> 4: Guilt feelings have become paranoid ideas.

## 8 Diminished Ability to Concentrate

Have you had any trouble concentrating or collecting your thoughts?

> Covers difficulties in concentration, making decisions about everyday matters.
>
> 0: Not present.
> 1: Very mild tendencies to concentration disturbances or problems in decision making.
> 2: Even with a major effort difficult to concentrate occasionally.
> 3: Difficulties in concentration even in things that usually need no effort (reading a newspaper, watching television program).
> 4: When it is clear that the patient is also showing difficulties in concentration during interview.

## 9 Recurrent Thoughts of Death, Suicidal Ideas or Plans

Have you had any thoughts that life is not worth living, or that you'd be better of dead? Would you prefer not to wake up tomorrow? What about thoughts of hurting or even killing yourself?

> Covers suicidal tendencies or plans. Is rated in degrees of probability of acting.
>
> 0: Not present.
> 1: The patient feels that life is not worthwhile, but expresses no wish to die.
> 2: The patient wishes to die but has no plans for taking his/her own life.
> 3: Probably has plans to hurt himself/herself.
> 4: Definitely has plans to kill himself/herself

# References

1. Bech P, Stage KB, Nair NPV et al. The Major Depression Rating Scale (MDS). Inter-rater reliability and validity across different settings in randomized moclobemide trials (submitted)
2. Stage KB (1996) Differences in symptomatology, diagnostic profile as well as adverse drug reactions between younger and elderly depressed patients. Thesis, Odense University
3. Williams JBW (1992) Structured interview guide for the HAM-D and MES. Biometrics Research Department, New York State Psychiatric Institute

# Appendix 4.
# Mastering Depression in Primary Care (MD/PC)

**Contents**

## 4.1 Introduction

The MASTERING system is an attempt to combine the WHO (Ten) Well-Being Questionnaire [1] and the WHO/ICD-10 criteria for depression [2] with the related Major Depression Rating Scale (ICD-10 version) to improve the recognition of major depression in general practice. MASTERING DEPRESSION stands for Measuring And Screening of Treatments Evaluated by Rating General practice Depression.

In Sect. 4.2 is shown a revised version of the WHO (Ten) Well-Being Questionnaire. The revision is a typographical division of the ten questions into five questions at the top and five questions at the bottom. This typographical revision gives the physician a quick scoring for screening depression analogue to PRIME-MD [3, 4]. The total score of the ten items would be used as an indicator of the general level of well-being, in itself a subjective outcome measure during treatment.

Section 4.3 shows how the physician should use the patient's scoring on the WHO Well-Being Questionnaire to measure the three symptoms of depression in ICD-10 referred to as B symptoms. If the patient has a yes (score 0 to 1) on two of the three B symptoms the physician proceeds to Sect. 4.4 for measuring the seven C symptoms which are the ultimate symptoms for diagnosing depression.

Section 4.4 shows how to arrive at a specific ICD-10 diagnosis of major depression on the basis of the B and C symptoms. Around 50% of patients with mild depression according to ICD-10 fulfills the criteria for major depression (F 32.0) [5].

Section 4.5 is the Major Depression Rating Scale modified for ICD-10. This modification involves a separation of the DSM-IV items of worthlessness and guilt into the item C4 (worthlessness) and item C5 (guilt).

In conclusion, Mastering Depression in Primary Care (MD-PC) is a three-stage procedure: Stage 1 is the screening questionnaire to be completed by the patient (WHO (Ten) Well-Being Questionnaire). Stage 2 is an application of the diagnostic criteria for DSM-IV major depression and ICD-10 depressive episode (F 32). Stage 3 is the outcome measure of treatment (Major Depression Rating Scale). This procedure is an example of parallel thinking in the patient-doctor collaboration [6].

## 4.2 WHO (Ten) Well-Being Questionnaire

*Please circle a number on each of the following <u>ten statements</u> to indicate how often you feel each of them has applied to you in the last <u>two weeks</u>.*

| PLEASE READ EACH OF THE STATEMENTS CAREFULLY | HIGHER SCORES MEAN BETTER WELL-BEING | | | |
|---|---|---|---|---|
| The first five statements are: | All of the time | More than half of the time | Less than half of the time | None of the time |
| 1 I feel downhearted and sad | 0 | 1 | 2 | 3 |
| 2 I feel calm and peaceful | 3 | 2 | 1 | 0 |
| 3 I feel energetic, active and vigorous | 3 | 2 | 1 | 0 |
| 4 I wake up feeling fresh and rested | 3 | 2 | 1 | 0 |
| 5 My daily life is full of things that were interest to me | 3 | 2 | 1 | 0 |
| The last five statements are: | All of the time | More than half of the time | Less than half of the time | None of the time |
| 6 I feel well adjusted to my life situation | 3 | 2 | 1 | 0 |
| 7 I live the kind of life I wanted | 3 | 2 | 1 | 0 |
| 8 I feel eager to tackle my daily tasks or make new decisions | 3 | 2 | 1 | 0 |
| 9 I feel I can easily handle or cope with any serious problem or major change in my life | 3 | 2 | 1 | 0 |
| 10 I am happy, satisfied or pleased with my personal life | 3 | 2 | 1 | 0 |

**Sub Total (first five statements)**  ☐☐

**Sub Total (last five statements)**  ☐☐

**Total (Ten) score**  ☐☐

## 4.3 WHO/ICD-10 Depressive Episode: Criteria A and B

**Criterion A** The statements or symptoms (see criteria B and C) should have lasted at least two weeks most of the time, e.g.: a score of 0 to 1 on the WHO (Ten) Well-Being Scale.

**Criterion B** Includes three symptoms (B1 Depressed mood; B2 Decreased energy; B3 Loss of interest). With reference to the WHO (Ten) Well-Being Scale the procedure is:

*"In the WHO questionnaire you said that..."*

If the patient has scored 0 to 1 on item 1: "That means that for most of the time you have been depressed"?

B1: Depressed mood    ☐ no   ☐ yes

If the patient has scored 0 to 1 on either item 3 or 4: "That means that most of the time you have had low energy"?

B2: Decreased energy    ☐ no   ☐ yes

If the patient has scored 0 to 1 on item 5: "That means that most of the time you have no interest in things"?

B3: Loss of interest    ☐ no   ☐ yes

If at least two boxes with "yes", go to Criterion C.

## 4.4 WHO/ICD-10 Depressive Episode: Criterion C

**Criterion C** covers the following C symptoms.

*For the last two weeks, have you had any of the following symptoms most of the time?*

|                                                                                   | No | Yes |
|-----------------------------------------------------------------------------------|----|-----|
| C1. Poor appetite and/or weight loss?                                             | ☐  | ☐   |
| C2. Trouble sleeping nearly every night?                                          | ☐  | ☐   |
| C3. Talk or move more slowly than normal, or restless more than usual?            | ☐  | ☐   |
| C4. Low self-confidence or worthlessness?                                         | ☐  | ☐   |
| C5. Feelings of self-reproach or guilt?                                           | ☐  | ☐   |
| C6. Diminished ability to concentrate?                                            | ☐  | ☐   |
| C7. Recurrent thoughts of death?                                                  | ☐  | ☐   |

Total number of "yes": ☐

## 4.5 WHO/ICD-10 Depression Diagnosis and DSM-IV Major Depression

| SYMPTOMS | yes = 1 no = 0 | F 32.0 Mild depression | F 32.1 Moderate depression | F 32.2 Severe depression |
|---|---|---|---|---|
| $B_1$ Depressed mood $B_2$ Decreased energy $B_3$ Loss of interest | ☐ ☐ ☐ | Two boxes with "yes" | Two boxes with "yes" | Three boxes with "yes" |
| $C_1$ Poor appetite or weight loss $C_2$ Insomnia $C_3$ Psychomotor retardation or agitation $C_4$ Worthlessness $C_5$ Guilt $C_6$ Diminished ability to concentrate $C_7$ Suicidal thoughts | ☐ ☐ ☐ ☐ ☐ ☐ ☐ | Two boxes with "yes" | Four boxes with "yes" | Five boxes with "yes" |
| Total B1−C7: Major depression | | Five boxes with "yes" | Five boxes with "yes" | Five boxes with "yes" |

## 4.6 Major Depression Rating Scale: ICD-10 Version

|  |  | Score |
|---|---|---|
| 1 Depressed mood | (0−4) | |
| 2 Diminished interests in social activities | (0−4) | |
| 3 Decreased appetite and/or significant weight loss (sum of 3a und 3b)<br><br>3a Decreased appetite (0−2)<br>3b Weight loss (0−2) | (0−4) | |
| 4 Insomnia | (0−4) | |
| 5 Psychomotor retardation and/or agitation (highest score on 5a and 5b)<br><br>5a Retardation (0−4)<br>5b Agitation (0−4) | (0−4) | |
| 6 Fatigue or loss of energy | (0−4) | |
| 7 Feelings of worthlessness and/or guilt (highest score on 7a or 7b)<br><br>7a Loss of self-esteem (0−4)<br>7b Guilt (0−4) | (0−4) | |
| 8 Diminished ability to concentrate | (0−4) | |
| 9 Recurrent thoughts of death, suicidal ideations or plans | (0−4) | |
| Total | (0−36) | |

# 4.7 Item Definitions

## General Remarks

The interview should assess the presence and intensity of the nine items one a minimum period of three days.

---

**1 Depressed mood**
Covers verbal and non-verbal communication of sadness, despair, despondency, helplessness and hopelessness.

0: Not present.
1: Very mild tendencies to lowered spirits.
2: The patient is more clearly concerned by unpleasant experiences although he or she still lacks feelings of hopelessness.
3: Moderately to markedly depressed. Some hopelessness and/or clear non-verbal signs of depression.
4: Severe degree of lowered mood. Pronounced hopelessness.

---

**2 Diminished interests in social activities**
Should be rated in degree of efficiency in social life functioning vs.: feels time usefully spend.

0: No difficulties; time feels useful.
1: Mild insufficiencies in social life activities; patient feels that he/she does not do enough with social life activities.
2: Clear (not up to standards) but still only moderate insufficiencies in the patient's day-to-day activities.
3: Difficulties in performing even daily routine activities, which are carried out with great efforts.
4: Often needs help in performing self care activities (unable to function independently).

---

**3 Decreased appetite and/or significant weight loss**

3a Decreased appetite
0: Not present.
1: Food intake is about or slightly less than normal; but without relish or tasteless.
2: Food intake is significantly reduced.

3b Weight loss
0: No weight loss.
1: Weight loss of 0.5 kg per week (or 1−2.5 in the current depressive episode).
2: Weight loss of 1 kg or more per week (or 3 kg or more in the current episode).

---

**4 Insomnia**

0: Usual sleep duration.
1: Duration of sleep slightly reduced.
2: Duration of sleep clearly reduced but still moderate, i.e., still less than a 50% reduction.
3: Duration of sleep markedly reduced.
4: Duration of sleep extremely reduced, e.g. as if had not been sleeping at all.

**5   Psychomotor retardation and/or agitation**

5a Retardation
0: Not present.
1: Conversational speed doubtfully or slightly reduced and facial expression doubtfully or slightly stiffened (retarded).
2: Conversational speed clearly reduced, with intermissions; reduced gestures and slow pace.
3: The interview is clearly prolonged due to long latencies and brief answers; all movements are very slow.
4: The interview cannot be completed; retardation approaches (and includes) stupor.

5b Agitation
0: Not present.
1: Doubtful or slight agitation, e.g. tendency to change position in chair or at times scratch his head.
2: Fidgeting; wringing hands, clearly changing position in chair now and again; clearly, but still moderately restless in ward, with some pacing.
3: Patient cannot stay in chair during interview (and/or much pacing in ward).
4: Interview must be conducted 'on the run'. Almost continuous pacing; pulling off clothes, tearing his hair.

**6   Fatigue or loss of energy**

0: Not present.
1: Very mild feelings of tiredness.
2: The patient is more clearly in a state of tiredness and weakness, but these symptoms are still without influence on the patient's daily life.
3: Marked feelings of tiredness which interfere occasionally with the patient's daily life.
4: Extreme feelings of tiredness interfering more constantly with the patient's daily life.

**7   Feelings of worthlessness and/or guilt**
Covers negative self-esteem and/or guilt feelings.

7a Worthlessness
0: Not present.
1: Slightly decreased self-confidence in relation to habitual level of social functioning.
2: Anticipates discomfort and failure in social relationships but still only to a moderate degree.
3: Is overconcerned about his/her standard of functioning compared to the standard of others, marked self-depreciation. Is clearly convinced emotionally of very poor functioning in usual activities but can intellectually still see that this view is unfounded.
4: Ideas of worthlessness have delusional, nihilistic degrees, i.e. cannot be corrected.

7b Guilt
0: Not present.
1: Concerned with the fact of being a burden to the family, friends or colleagues due to reduced interests in usual activities.
2: Guilt feelings are clearly present because the patient is concerned with incidents (minor omissions or failures) in the past prior to the current episode of depression.
3: Feelings that current depression is a punishment but can still see intellectually that this view is unfounded.
4: Guilt feelings have become paranoid ideas.

---

**8  Diminished ability to concentrate**
Covers difficulties in concentration, making decisions about everyday matters.

0: Not present.
1: Very mild tendencies of concentration disturbances or problems in decision making.
2: Even with a major effort difficult to concentrate occasionally.
3: Difficulties in concentration even in things that usually need no effort (reading a newspaper, watching television program).
4: When it is clear that the patient during interview is also showing difficulties in concentration.

---

**9  Recurrent thoughts of death, suicidal ideations or plans**
Covers suicidal tendencies or plans. Is rated in degrees of probability of acting.

0: Not present.
1: The patient feels that life is not worthwhile, but expresses no wish to die.
2: The patient wishes to die but has no plans of taking his/her own life.
3: Probably has active plans to hurt himself/herself.
4: Definitely has plans to kill himself/herself.

---

# References

1. Bech P, Staehr Johansen K, Gudex C (1996) The WHO (Ten) Well-Being Index: Validation in diabetes. Psychotherapy and Psychosomatics (in press)
2. World Health Organization (1993) The ICD-10 classification of mental and behavioural disorders. Diagnostic criteria for research. World Health Organization, Geneva
3. Spitzer RL, Williams JBW, Kroenke K et al. (1994) Utility of a new procedure for diagnosing mental disorders in primary care: the PRIME-MD 1000 study. JAMA 272:1749–1756
4. Broadhead EW, Leon AC, Weissman MM et al. (1995) Development and validation of the SDDS-PC screen for multiple mental disorders in primary care. Arch Fam med 4:211–219
5. Bertelsen A (1995) Personal communication. November, 1995
6. de Bono E (1994) Parallel thinking. Viking, London

# Appendix 5.
# DSM-IV Manic State Rating Scale

**Contents**

| ITEM | | | Score |
|------|------|------|-------|
| A | Mood (highest score) <br><br> A1 Elevated mood $(0-4)$ <br> A2 Irritable mood $(0-4)$ | $(0-4)$ | |
| B | B1 Increased self-esteem | $(0-4)$ | |
| | B2 Sleep disturbances | $(0-4)$ | |
| | B3 Talkativeness | $(0-4)$ | |
| | B4 Flight of ideas | $(0-4)$ | |
| | B5 Distractability | $(0-4)$ | |
| | B6 Activities (highest score) <br><br> a Social contacts $(0-4)$ <br> b Psychomotor $(0-4)$ | $(0-4)$ | |
| | B7 Risk taking behaviour | $(0-4)$ | |
| | Total | $(0-32)$ | |

## 5.2 Item Definitions

### General Remarks

The interview should assess the presence and intensity of the eight items over a minimum period of three days.

### A1 Elevated mood

0: Not present.
1: Slightly elevated mood, optimistic, but still adapted to situation.
2: Moderately elevated mood, joking, laughing, however, somewhat irrelevant to situation.
3: Markedly elevated mood, exuberant both in manner and speech, clearly irrelevant to situation.
4: Extremely elevated mood, quite irrelevant to situation.

## A2   Irritable mood

0:   Not present.
1:   Somewhat impatient or irritable, but control is maintained.
2:   Moderately impatient or irritable. Does not tolerate provocations.
3:   Provocative, makes threats, but can be calmed down.
4:   Overt physical violence; physical destructive.

## B1   Increased self-esteem

0:   Not present.
1:   Slightly increased self-esteem, for example, overestimates slightly own habitual capabilities.
2:   Moderately increased self-esteem, for example, overestimates more clearly own habitual capabilities or hints at unusual abilities.
3:   Markedly unrealistic ideas, for example, believes he/she possesses extraordinary abilities, powers or knowledge (scientific, religious etc.), but can quickly be corrected.
4:   Grandiose ideas which cannot be corrected.

## B2   Sleep disturbances

This item covers the patient's subjective experience of the duration of sleep (hours of sleep per 24-h periods). The rating should be based on the three preceding nights, irrespective of the administration of hypnotics or sedatives. The score is the average of the past three nights.

0:   Not present (habitual duration of sleep).
1:   Duration of sleep reduced by 25%.
2:   Duration of sleep reduced by 50%.
3:   Duration of sleep reduced by 75%.
4:   No sleep.

## B3   Talkativeness (pressure of speech)

0:   Not present.
1:   Somewhat talkative.
2:   Clearly talkative, few spontaneous intervals in the conversation, but still not difficult to interrupt.
3:   Almost no spontaneous intervals in the conversation, difficult to interrupt.
4:   Impossible to interrupt, dominates the conversation completely.

## B4   Flight of thoughts

0:   Not present.
1:   Somewhat lively in descriptions, explanations and elaborations without losing the connection with the topic of the conversation. The thoughts are thus still coherent.

2: The patient's thoughts are occasionally distracted by random associations (often rhymes, slangs, puns, pieces of verse or music).
3: The line of thought is more regularly disrupted by diversionary associations.
4: It is very difficult or impossible to follow the patient because of the flight of thoughts; he or she constantly jumps from one topic to another.

## B5 Distractability

Social activity should be measured in terms of the degree of disability or distractability in social, occupational or other important areas of functioning.

0: No difficulties.
1: Slightly increased drive, but work quality is slightly reduced as motivation is changing; the patient is somewhat distractible (attention drawn to irrelevant stimuli).
2: Work activity clearly affected by distractability, but still to a moderate degree.
3: The patient occasionally loses control of routine tasks because of marked distractability.
4: Unable to perform any task without help.

## B6 Activities

### a Social Contacts
0: Not present.
1: Slightly meddling (putting his/her oar in), slightly intrusive.
2: Moderately meddling and arguing or intrusive.
3: Dominating, arranging, directing, but still in contact with the setting.
4: Extremely dominating.

### b Psychomotor
0: Not present.
1: Slightly increased motor activity (e.g. some tendency to lively facial expression).
2: Clearly increased motor activity (e.g. lively facial expression, not able to sit quietly in chair).
3: Excessive motor activity, on the move most of the time, but the patient can sit still if urged to (rises only once during interview).
4: Constantly active, restlessly energetic. Even if urged to, the patient cannot sit still.

## B7 Risk taking behaviour

This item covers excessive involvement in pleasurable activities that have a high potential for painful consequences (e.g. engaging in unrestrained buying sprees, sexual indiscretions, or foolish business investments).

0: Not present.
1: Slight risk taking behaviour.
2: Moderate risk taking behaviour.
3: Marked risk taking behaviour.
4: Extreme risk taking behaviour.

# Appendix 6.
# The Calgary Depression Scale for Schizophrenia (CDSS)

**Contents**

## 6.1 Scoring Sheet

| No. | Item | | Score |
|-----|------|------|-------|
| 1 | Depressed mood | (0−3) | |
| 2 | Hopelessness | (0−3) | |
| 3 | Self depreciation | (0−3) | |
| 4 | Guilty ideas of reference | (0−3) | |
| 5 | Pathological guilt | (0−3) | |
| 6 | Morning depression | (0−3) | |
| 7 | Early wakening | (0−3) | |
| 8 | Suicide | (0−3) | |
| 9 | Observed depression | (0−3) | |
| | Total score | (0−27) | |

## 6.2 Item Definitions

### General Remarks

The interviewer should ask the first question as written. Use follow up probes or qualifiers at your discretion. Time frame refers to last two weeks unless stipulated. It should be emphasized that item 9 is based on observations of the entire interview.

## Item Specifications

### Item 1   Depression
How would you describe your mood over the last two weeks:
Do you keep reasonably cheerful or have you been very depressed or low
spirited recently? In the last two weeks how often have you (own words) every
day? All day?

0:   Absent
1:   Mild          Expresses some sadness or discouragement on questioning.
2:   Moderate      Distinct depressed mood persisting up to half the time over
                   last 2 weeks: present daily.
3:   Severe        Markedly depressed mood persisting daily over half the time
                   interfering with normal motor and social functioning.

### Item 2   Hopelessness
How do you see the future for yourself?
Can you see any future? − or has life seemed quite hopeless?
Have you given up or does there still seem some reason for trying?

0:   Absent
1:   Mild          Has at times felt hopeless over the last week but still has some
                   degree of hope for the future.
2:   Moderate      Persistent, moderate sense of hopelessness over last week.
                   Can be persuaded to acknowledge possibility of things being
                   better.
3:   Severe        Persisting and distressing sense of hopelessness.

### Item 3   Self depreciation
What is your opinion of yourself compared to other people?
Do you feel better, not as good, or about the same as other?
Do you feel inferior or even worthless?

0:   Absent
1:   Mild          Some inferiority; not amounting to feeling of worthlessness.
2:   Moderate      Subject feels worthless, but less than 50% of the time.
3:   Severe        Subject feels worthless more than 50% of the time. May be
                   challenged to acknowledge otherwise.

### Item 4   Guilty ideas of reference
Do you have the feeling that you are being blamed for something or even
wrongly accused? What about? (do not include justifiable blame or accusa-
tion. Exclude delusions of guilt).

0:   Absent
1:   Mild          Subject feels blamed but not accused less than 50% of the
                   time.

| 2: | Moderate | Persisting sense of being blamed, and/or occasional sense of being accused. |
|----|----------|------------------|
| 3: | Severe | Persistent sense of being accused. When challenged, acknowledges that it is *not* so. |

### Item 5  Pathological guilt

Do you tend to blame yourself for little things you may have done in the past?
Do you think that you deserve to be so concerned about this?

| 0: | Absent | |
|----|--------|------------------|
| 1: | Mild | Subject sometimes feels over guilty about some minor peccadillo, but less than 50% of time. |
| 2: | Moderate | Subject usually (over 50% of time) feels guilty about past actions the significance of which he/she exaggerates. |
| 3: | Severe | Subject usually feels she/he is to blame for everything that has gone wrong, even when not his/her fault. |

### Item 6  Morning depression

When you have felt depressed over the last 2 weeks have you noticed the depression being worse at any particular time of day?

| 0: | Absent | No depression. |
|----|--------|------------------|
| 1: | Mild | Depression present but no diurnal variation. |
| 2: | Moderate | Depression spontaneously mentioned to be worse in a.m. |
| 3: | Severe | Depression markedly worse in a.m., with impaired functioning which improves in p.m. |

### Item 7  Early wakening

Do you wake earlier in the morning than is normal for you?
How many times a week does this happen?

| 0: | Absent | |
|----|--------|------------------|
| 1: | Mild | Occasionally wakes (up to twice weekly) 1 hour or more before normal time to wake or alarm time. |
| 2: | Moderate | Often wakes early (up to 5 times weekly) 1 hour or more before normal time to wake or alarm. |
| 3: | Severe | Daily wakes 1 hour or more before normal time. |

### Item 8  Suicide

Have you felt that life wasn't worth living? Did you ever feel like ending it all?
What did you think you might do? Did you actually try?

| 0: | Absent | |
|----|--------|------------------|
| 1: | Mild | Frequent thoughts of being better off dead, or occasional thoughts of suicide. |
| 2: | Moderate | Deliberately considered suicide with a plan, but made no attempt. |

3: Severe        Suicidal attempt apparently designed to end in death (i.e.: accidental discovery or inefficient means).

**Item 9    Observed depression**
Based on interviewer's observations during the entire interview.
The question "Do you feel like crying?" used at appropriate points in the interview, may elicit information useful to this observation.

0: Absent
1: Mild          Subject appears sad and mournful even during parts of the interview, involving affectively neutral discussion.
2: Moderate   Subject appears sad and mournful throughout the interview, with gloomy monotonous voice and is tearful or close to tears at times.
3: Severe       Subject chokes on distressing topics, frequently sighs deeply and cries openly, or is persistently in a state of frozen misery if examiner is sure that this is present.

## 6.3 Psychometric Description

*Type:* Symptom scale.

*Subject area:* Assessment of depressive symptoms separate from positive, negative and extrapyramidal symptoms in people with schizophrenia.

*Administration:* Observer scale. Semi-structured, goal-directed interview.

*Time axis:* Previous two weeks unless otherwise specified.

*Item selection:* Factor analysis of the Present State Examination and the HAM-D [1].

*Number of items:* Nine.

*Definition of items:* All items are defined according to operational criteria from 0 to 3.

*Psychometric validity:* The internal validity of the scale has been verified by use of confirmative factor analysis as well as Cronbach's alpha coefficient [2]. Compared to HAM-D the CDSS has higher degree of discriminant validity in diagnosing depression in schizophrenic patients, i.e. a high specificity [3, 4].

**Comments**

The high ability of the CDSS to measure depression in schizophrenic patients has recently been confirmed [5], i.e. lack of correlation to positive or negative symptoms of schizophrenia as well as extrapyramidal symptoms induced by neuroleptic treatment. The applicability of the CDSS is superior to self-rating scales for depression (the Beck Depression Inventory) emphasizing that observer scales are recommended in the population of schizophrenic patients [6].

Those who want to know more about the CDSS should contact its architect, Dr. D. Addington, Dept. of Psychiatry, Foothills Hospital, Calgary, Alberta T2N 2T9, Canada.

# References

1. Addington D, Addington J, Schissel B (1990) A depression rating scale for depression. Schizophrenia Research 3:247–251
2. Addington D, Addington J, Matricka-Tyndale E, Joyce J (1992) Reliability and validity of a depression rating scale for schizophrenics. Schizophrenia Research 6:201–208
3. Addington D, Addington J, Matricka-Tyndale E (1994) Specificity of the Calgary Depression Scale for schizophrenia. Schizophrenia Research 11:239–244
4. Addington D, Addington J, Matricka-Tyndale E (1993) Assessing depression in schizophrenia: The Calgary Depression Scale. Br J Psychiat 163 (Suppl 22):39–44
5. Addington D, Addington J, Atkinson M (1996) A psychometric comparison of the Calgary Depression Scale for Schizophrenia and the Hamilton Depression Rating Scale. Schizophrenia Research (in press)
6. Addington D, Addington J, Matricka-Tyndale E (1993) Rating depression in schizophrenia. A comparison of a self-report and an observer report scale. J Nerv Ment Dis 181:561–565

# 7 Epilogue

This twenty years update of the Hamilton Depression Scale (HAM-D) has via the Bech-Rafaelsen Melancholia Scale (MES) resulted in the Major Depression Rating Scale (MDS) with reference both to DSM-IV and ICD-10. Likewise, the Mania Scale (MAS) has been developed into the DSM-IV Manic State Rating Scale.

The twenty years update of the Zung Self-rating Depression Scale (ZUNG-D) has resulted in a WHO Well-Being Questionnaire, the WHO (Ten) scale.

An integration of the WHO (Ten) Well-Being Questionnaire and the Major Depression Rating Scale has been outlined as the MASTERING DEPRESSION. The idea of combining a patient questionnaire with a clinician interview is also used in PRIME-MD [1]. Another example is the PCASEE questionnaire (constructed as a health-related quality of life scale) and, on the one hand, the individual quality of life computer version [2], or, on the other hand, the Major Depression Rating Scale. In other words, a quality of life questionnaire can be supplemented either with a more deep interview for quality of life or with a scale for major depression. The screening of depression is essentially a screening for quality of life [3, 4]: is life worth living?

The complete picture of mood disorders ("major affective disorders") includes both mania and aggression. The attempt to update the Bech-Rafaelsen Mania Scale has resulted in a new, supplemental, scale, the Social Dysfunction and Aggression Scale (SDAS). Both scales are often needed when measuring outcomes of elevated mood disorders.

The references to DSM-IV and ICD-10 are references to classification systems without proper quantification, i.e. dichotomies. In contrast, rating scales are quantifying mood disorders in a naturalistic and empirical meaningful way: They are non-dichotomies or pluralistic [5]. Furthermore, an example of a depression scale developed to capture mood symptoms in schizophrenia has been included [6].

In Europe ICD-10 is the official diagnostic system although the DSM-IV diagnosis of major depression is the conventional indication of antidepressant drugs. In Table 3 are shown the ICD-10 codes for depressive episodes with reference to major depression, atypical or masked depression and melancholia at the level of the fourth character of F 32. – . At the etiological level (endogenous depression) the ICD-10 codes refer to the somatic syndrome [7], which is used for the mild and moderate degree to confirm the use of antidepressant drugs in cases where major depression is uncertain. Throughout this book we have equalled major depression with moderate depression and melancholia with the Hippocratic tradition to denote generally the depressive (unspecified) syndrome [8]. The most important fact clinically about melancholia or depression is that we can measure it and treat it with antidepressant drugs.

**Table 3.** Depressive Episode: ICD-10/F32. –

```
Fourth character: –
0:  mild (F 32.0)      ⎫
1:  moderate (F 32.1)  ⎬  major depression (see Appendix 4); endogenous depression
                       ⎭
2:  severe, without psychotic symptoms
3:  severe, with psychotic symptoms
8:  other (atypical, masked)
9:  unspecified (melancholia)
```

Fifth character: –
0: without somatic syndrome (F 32.x0)  ⎫
1: with somatic syndrome (F 32.x1)     ⎬  (see Diagnostic Melancholia Scale)
                                       ⎭

# References

1. Spitzer RL, Williams JBW, Kroenke K et al (1994) Utility of a new procedure for diagnosing mental disorders in primary care: The PRIME-MD 1000 study. JAMA 272: 1749–1756
2. Thunedborg K, Black C, Bech P (1995) Beyond the Hamilton Depression Scores in the long-term treatment of manic-melancholic patients: Prediction of recurrence of depression by quality of life measurements. Psychotherapy and Psychosomatics 64:131–140
3. Bech P (1995) Rating scales to evaluate quality of life of depressed patients. WPA Teaching Bulletin 3:1–3
4. James W (1902) The varieties of religious experience. Longmans, London
5. James W (1909) A pluralistic universe. Longmans, London
6. Addington D, Addington J, Schissel B (1990) A depression rating scale for schizophrenics. Schizophrenia Research 3:247–251
7. World Health Organization (1992) The ICD-10 classification of mental and behavioural disorders. Clinical descriptions. World Health Organization, Geneva
8. World Health Organization (1994) Lexicon of psychiatric and mental health terms. World Health Organization, Geneva

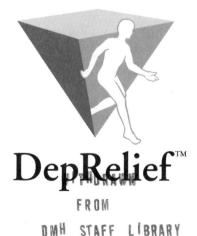

DepRelief™

FROM

DMH STAFF LIBRARY

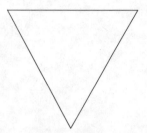

Internal validity

Inter-rater reliability

External validity

**Springer**
*Berlin*
*Heidelberg*
*New York*
*Barcelona*
*Budapest*
*Hong Kong*
*London*
*Milan*
*Paris*
*Santa Clara*
*Singapore*
*Tokyo*